Renegade Patient

Renegade Patient

The No-Nonsense, Practical Guide to Getting the Health Care You Need

By **Tedde Rinker, D.O.**

Foreword by
Parris M. Kidd, Ph.D.

BioMed Publishing Group

BioMed Publishing Group
P.O. Box 9012
South Lake Tahoe, CA 96158
www.LymeBook.com

ISBN 10: 0-9763797-7-5
ISBN 13: 978-0-9763797-7-5

For related books and DVDs visit us online at www.lymebook.com.

Disclaimer

This book is not intended as medical advice. It is also not intended to prevent, diagnose, treat or cure disease. Instead, the book is intended only to share the author's research, as would an investigative journalist. The book is provided for informational and educational purposes only, not as treatment instructions for any disease. If you have a medical problem, please make an appointment with a licensed physician.

To purchase additional copies of this book or to place orders in wholesale quantity, visit www.biomedpublishers.com.

Visit the author's website at www.stress-medicine.com.

Table of Contents

Acknowledgements

This book has been a process for me, supported and inspired by many people. My great friend, colleague, and mentor, Parris Kidd, was an enthusiastic supporter from the very first conversations about a book with this concept, in support of patient's independence. He, along with Bruce Janke and Raymonde Guindon, were my first readers, who gave me valuable feedback on my writing approach. I am very grateful to Helena Milligan who helped me prepare my first draft to present to publishers, and to Julie Byers, who helped with the final polishing, editing and furniture rearranging to get it to the completed version before you. Bryan Rosner, my publisher, is also a great writer whose style inspired me to believe that my conversational style of writing may have some appeal. I had help with patient and professional interviews from Liam Satre-Melloy, who was able to travel to places I wasn't to get stories from several people around the country. Thanks to Deborah Beale for her guidance in the process of finding and working with a publisher.

There are many great and inspiring health care providers, whom I consider mentors. I can't name them all here, but some of them, who would be considered "renegade doctors" by the more conventional medical community, give their time and energy to teach other health care providers to look at more than just the "chief complaint" and to do more than hand out a prescription. Some of these are: David Perlmutter, a great writer and teacher (who has a blog entitled Renegade Neurologist), Neal Rouzier, a brave and brilliant teacher about natural (bio-identical hormone) replacement, and Denis Wilson and Michael Freidman of Wilson Temperature Syndrome, who teach physicians and patients that thyroid function can be greatly improved and restored to normal. Patrick Hanaway of Genova Diagnostics, helping healthcare providers understand how to use laboratory data to move a patient toward great health and disease prevention. Dharma

Singh Kahlsa, one of the first physicians in America to speak out and teach others about preventing dementia, and Robert Goldman and Ronald Klatz, for founding the American Academy of Anti-Aging Medicine, now a worldwide organization dedicated to teaching preventive medicine, slowing degenerative diseases of aging, and ultimately lengthening the healthy human lifespan. While anti-aging medicine has triggered controversy, there is no doubt that their work has profoundly influenced the direction of research and broadened the goals of thousands of healthcare providers, to include helping patients feel vital, strong and healthy, well into their senior years.

I want to thank the patients who were willing to share their stories. Some of them requested that I change their identifying characteristics, because they had fear of retaliation from healthcare providers or insurance companies. I have done so. If you recognize a name or think you know this person, chances are you don't. I thank also all of the patients I have worked with over the years for what they have taught me. I have learned much from those who had learned the hard way that they had to be "tough" to get what they needed and wanted from the medical system. I gladly share their wisdom with you. I thank my family for their love and for the joy they bring me; my children, Gaia and Max, and Larry, my spouse, my beloved, and my best friend.

Finally, I would like to thank Scott Forsgren, a "renegade patient role model," who reviewed the book prior to publication and provided a number of helpful suggestions.

Foreword by Parris M. Kidd, PhD

Welcome to the world of the empowered patient. This book teaches us as "healthcare consumers" how to deal effectively with the healthcare system, to get from it what it's supposed to give us—better health. This is a rare gem of a book, because it lays bare the workings of the healthcare system that consumers normally are not allowed to know. And it is written not by a consumer advocate, but by a healthcare insider—a doctor.

Tedde Rinker is that rare physician who truly listens to her patients. She sincerely wants her patients to recover from their illness, not just go home with a purple pill. She is a highly experienced and versatile physician, thoroughly familiar with the problems of the existing healthcare system, and here she gives us the info we so desperately need to make the system work for us. She also informs her physician colleagues how to make the system work better for them while doing better for their patients.

The central reality that drove Dr. Rinker to do this book is that the healthcare system is driven more by money and profit than it is by compassion for the patient. She speaks to the reader not just as a physician but also as a patient herself. As a guiding theme for the book, she unveils a Declaration of Independence for Health Care. This alone makes the book worth reading, and should be given a place of prominence in every household in the world.

Dr. Rinker also gets down to the nitty gritty of medical practice, and what the sick person could expect to get from caring healthcare providers. A lot of people have illness that doesn't fit into the conventional diagnostic categories. This has more to do with the outmoded approach to diagnosis than it does with patients imagining illness or trying to "game" the system. This book is focused where the mainstream is most out of focus—on helping the patient as a whole and deserving individual. On safe, curative, integrative medical practice as opposed to doling out the newest drugs with often-undisclosed side effects. On helping the body to heal itself.

All of us in the Western world are raised to worship doctors. Whatever our doctor tells us to do, we do. After all, the doctor has been to medical school and we are only patients. Dr. Rinker has the courage to remind us that our doctor isn't always right. After all, we are living in our bodies, not the doctor. Our bodies belong to us, and we're responsible for our health. This means you need to get your doctor to accept you as a partner in the project to make you well.

But physicians increasingly are being limited by the system in what they can do for their patients. Today's practitioner is under incredible pressure from overhead costs—liability insurance, equipment, restrictions from the insurance companies, and pressure from the medical boards to stick to mediocre practice of medicine. Rather than demonize the doc, better that we understand their limitations and help them to help us. And sometimes we'll have to pay outside the insurance system to get that healing treatment insurance won't pay for.

Dr. Rinker also has done well for us by avoiding health fads. There's no 7-day diet in these pages. There are no miracle cures, no quick fixes. To the contrary, she gives a balanced explanation of CAM (Complementary and Alternative Medicine) in its many forms. This reminded me how acupuncture, chiropractic, and dietary supplements helped me recover from a bad fall—they were the only things that helped. She covers the diversity of CAM healing systems that existed long before the Western system, and gives useful information on the many types of healthcare practitioners trained to use them. She even gives tips on how to obtain your records, and formats for how to organize them!

We have the right to caring and competent (and yes, affordable) health care. This means making ourselves more educated about health and how the body works. This book is generous with resources for healthcare information. The reader should take advantage of these, because to survive the system we need to ask a lot of questions. We need to keep our own complete sets of records, become fully informed about our particular health problems, research controversial issues, and so become fully equipped to represent our needs when that becomes necessary. The book urges readers to develop a "healthy skepticism" when dealing with their health. Some may call us renegades, but we'll survive better than those who don't assert their needs.

Because, let's face it, just dealing with the healthcare system is a struggle for survival. Physically, mentally, emotionally, spiritually, financially, the system can crush the unsuspecting patient. Dispensing synthetic hormones to women. Misrepresenting toxic drugs as being safe. Manipulating public opinion against non-pharmacologic medical practice. Failing to enforce food safety regulations. Gouging healthcare premiums to profit from our suffering. This book brilliantly helps us navigate the system to get the help we need for our health. Enjoy this book and feel your power.

Parris M. Kidd, PhD

www.DocKidd.com

Author of "Phosphatidyl Serine: Nature's Brain Booster" and "GlycerPhosphoCholine: Mind-Body Power for Active Living and Healthy Aging"

Author's Preface

If you are a consumer of health care—as we all are at one time or another—you know the system is not perfect. The technology is there, and so are well trained and highly skilled medical professionals, yet the picture is far from pretty.

As patients, we frequently are putty in the hands of doctors, health insurance companies, and the pharmaceutical industry. We are caught in a system driven by profits, rather than by genuine and selfless concern for the physical, mental, and emotional well-being of a patient.

The culture of mainstream medicine is a closed system, constrained by insurance companies and controlled largely by powerful drug manufacturers who spend *billions* each year marketing their product to both physicians and the public.

In this flawed context *you*, the consumer, lose out, while the medical industry is the big winner.

How to remedy this? In order to regain the advantage, you must be willing to assume responsibility for managing your own health care, by becoming an active and informed participant in your quest for good health.

In short, you must become your own health care advocate. This may sound like a daunting task, and sometimes it is. But your health is undeniably your most precious commodity, and no effort should be spared in protecting it.

How should you go about becoming an empowered advocate of your own health care?

Whether you are an impassioned activist or are just interested in learning how to protect yourself, this book will give you useful information, resources, examples, real-life testimonials, and inspiration to take charge of the most important commodity you have.

Before you start reading

Although the U.S. Advisory Commission on Consumer Protection adopted the Patient's Bill of Rights in 1998 (examined more closely in Chapter 3 of this book), it has not fundamentally changed the way health care providers respond to patient needs. As a result, I saw the need to create my own patient manifesto, written from the perspective of patients who have freed themselves from passive compliance with traditional medical dictates.

Our country was founded on the Declaration of Independence, right? Here is the Declaration of Independence for Health Care, summarizing the principles in this book. I have carefully formulated this declaration through years of experience in medical practice and careful observation of medical care in the United States. These guidelines serve as cornerstone principles in my medical practice. The majority of health care providers will neither be aware of these points nor support them, so each of us must individually pursue these rights in order to obtain their benefits. It is all in your hands.

Declaration of Independence for Health Care

We the people, being of sound mind and independent spirit, do hereby declare our freedom from the domination of modern myths that keep us from attaining optimal health:

1. We reject the myth that the doctor has all the answers. We no longer accept "orders" from physicians. We expect to be treated as equals and to have any proposed diagnoses or treatments explained fully, to our satisfaction and complete

understanding. We expect courteous treatment and cooperation if and when we decide a second opinion is warranted.

2. We reject the myth that health insurance companies exist solely for the benefit of our health. We realize they are in business for their own profit. When we, and our health care providers, consider services medically necessary, but the insurance company deems them unneeded, we will protest. We will not let the profit motives of insurance carriers dictate what we will and will not do to achieve health.

3. We are skeptical of the pharmaceutical companies who control their own research and select only what they choose to reveal. We also refute the notion that all FDA approved drugs are safe and that the extraordinarily high price we pay for prescription medications is for research (when, in fact, most of it is earmarked for lobbying and marketing). We demand more accurate information about medication risks from both the pharmaceutical industry and the prescribing doctors. We also demand more accurate information from the Nutraceutical industry (defined as "food, or parts of food, that provide medical or health benefits, including the prevention and treatment of disease") about the risks, benefits, and actual content of the active ingredients in their products.

4. We reject the assumption that records relating to our health or illness are the property of the doctor or institution where we sought consultation or medical treatment. These records are ours by right, as they are personal and relevant to each of us as individuals. We demand the right to review these records at any time and to have copies of any medical records we deem important for our own personal files. We are also aware that we have the legal right to make corrections when incorrect information is present in a chart.

5. We reject not only the myth that there is only one legitimate or standard type of medical practice, but also the belief that the double-blind placebo-controlled study is the only method needed to determine an effective treatment. We expect a good physician to be aware of alternatives or to be willing to admit that he or she does not know of alternative treatments, so that we are able to determine for ourselves if we want to seek additional expert advice.

6. We do not believe that disability and fragile health are a natural consequence of aging. We will not settle for treatments that cover up our symptoms but do not reverse degenerative processes, especially when alternative treatments are available. We want to know when lifestyle and diet are critical factors for health-threatening illnesses. We do not want the physician to withhold this information believing that it is irrelevant.

7. We declare ourselves competent to make informed decisions about our health and well-being and want to be part of every decision concerning our health and recovery from illness. We want information. We want alternatives. We want to be at the center of the decision-making process. If a health care provider cannot agree to these stipulations, we want to be told, so that we may choose a different provider.

Use the seven points in this declaration as a guideline. Learn to pursue all your options. Use the references and templates provided in this book to compile your own medical record and negotiate a more active role in any treatment you consider or receive. Rate your health care professionals: the ones you like (especially) and the ones you think that you and others should avoid.

The internet is a valuable resource for the patient/consumer wanting to be better informed about medical choices. Fortunately, more and more of us have online access to medical information. The many websites I will mention in this book are not meant to be endorsements of any particular medical protocol, but are merely examples of what I found when I searched for solutions and resources. I certainly have not followed up with treatment at all the websites that offer information and referrals, and could not possibly endorse all the practitioners listed on these websites. They are merely examples of the wealth of information available when searching for solutions and resources. How to use them is for you to determine, using your own judgment.

Ready to become an informed, empowered patient?

Well then, let's go!

Chapter 1

How I Got Fed Up With The System

I am an Osteopathic physician (D.O.). As such, I practice a whole-person approach, which means I treat both the physical and mental needs of my patients. In the United States, Doctors of Osteopathic Medicine are fully licensed physicians and surgeons, practicing medicine in all clinical specialties. D.O.'s hold doctorates of medicine that are very similar to the degrees held by the far more common allopathic physicians (M.D.'s), and the training that the two professions receive is, in most ways, virtually identical.

I grew up one block away from an Osteopathic hospital in the Midwest, but my parents never used that facility for health care. Even when my father was dying from a ruptured aneurysm, he wanted the ambulance to take him to the "regular" hospital two miles away. As it turned out, no matter what choice he would have made or what kind of medical care he would have received, his life was over that day. Even today, 35 years later, there is nothing we can do for a ruptured aorta, as it is the biggest blood vessel in the body and is located very close to the heart.

However, for treating the great majority of medical conditions, we have a range of choices and treatment options which most people, like my own parents, don't know exist. I was 15-years-old at the time my father died and had yet made no conscious decision to become a physician. In fact, in college I changed my major several times, finally settling on medical school because I was fascinated with the human body and mind. My last major had been in environmental science, and I had begun to see that research in this field was being manipulated by politicians to serve non-ecological purposes. As an idealist, I decided I did not wish to be part of that unethical process. I wanted to keep on learning, and I made the decision to apply to medical schools.

I had worked in hospitals while attending college: drawing blood, assisting in the lab, and as a research assistant to an oncologist. I became acquainted with an Osteopathic physician who was doing a post-graduate fellowship in oncology with my M.D. boss. I was in the process of applying to medical schools at that time, and because of my family's bias (they believed—erroneously of course—that Osteopathic physicians were not "real doctors" and that they received inferior medical training), I had not considered applying to Osteopathic medical schools and knew nothing about them. The physician with whom I worked told me one thing that altered my thinking and made an indelible impression on me: the philosophy of Osteopathic medicine was, first and foremost, to assist the body to heal itself.

As an environmental science major, the idea of healing a human being within the system of his or her own body's resources made a lot of sense to me. So, I added four Osteopathic medical schools to the list of applications I sent out.

While I was awaiting an interview at one of the conventional medical schools on my list, Michigan State University's College of Osteopathic Medicine invited me for an interview. Following the meeting, I was offered a position in the entering class of 1975. Even though I was impressed with the Michigan State curriculum, I worried a little about the public's prejudice against Osteopathic physicians, the same kind of preconceptions my parents had. Still, I did not want to miss my chance to get into medical school, as the competition for the few spots reserved for women by "affirmative action" (which actually *reduced* the number of available seats) was fierce. I was eager to learn, so I accepted, and to this day, I have never regretted this decision.

The Osteopathic Medical school was everything it promised to be. I did learn about the whole body as an integrated, complex system. The subject of nutrition was sadly sparse, as it is in nearly all medical schools, but I learned a lot about the mechanics of the bones, muscles, nerves, lymphatic system, and the spine. I also learned how the knowledge and understanding of internal processes could facilitate and speed up healing. Last, but not least, when I later compared notes with my M.D. counterparts, I realized that my grasp of how the various body systems integrated with each other was better than theirs.

In the hospital setting, however, many of the principles we had been taught were not applied. Perhaps a more holistic diagnostic process was considered, because our training caused us to think in terms of system over specialty, but in practice, the D.O. hospital was almost identical to an M.D. hospital. This might have reassured my father, if he had ever bothered to look into the qualifications of various medical schools, but it disappointed me. I thought I would see the next–*higher*–level of applied integrated care.

I did not realize at first what was wrong with this picture. I thought at the time that most specialties would end up boring me. I would memorize a set of diagnostic cues within my specialty area, remember which tests should be done to elicit a diagnosis, as well as a few possible alternatives, then memorize the recommended treatments and prescribe them. I was a very enthusiastic student, but this process did nothing to encourage or motivate me. So, for my residency training, I chose the one specialty that seemed to offer the most intellectual flexibility: Psychiatry.

Many of my mentors were surprised by this choice, because they thought I was too bright to "leave medicine." But I saw the field of psychiatry, as it was in 1978, as one of the only frontiers left, where doctors did not have pat answers for everything. I believed there was still a lot to learn and to explore. It did not take too long, however, for my vision of that broad vista to narrow down to a very specific categorical classification of behaviors, thoughts, and feelings, which, in turn, developed into a diagnosis, with a few possible alternative diagnoses, and a list of suitable prescription medications. Boom, done.

Despite my dislike of the field's rigidity, helping people through psychotherapy was a privilege and an adventure. I only hope that I helped as much as I learned, because my heart and intellect were committed to my patients. I had never thought of the mind as being separate from the body or the body as separate from the mind. This belief guided my work as a psychiatrist in many ways, and still guides me today.

After my graduation and residency, I started an outpatient practice with a therapist partner. We named our clinic "Stress Medicine Consulting." Many of our patients were "outcasts" referred by other therapists and medical doctors. Mainstream physicians do not look kindly upon patients with psychosomatic symptoms, or with multiple symptoms in many organ systems.

Conventional doctors generally are uncomfortable with patients who complain of many different ailments. If emotions or stress cause physical symptoms, it is common for physicians to consider such symptoms as malingering. But these patients have real pain, real fear, and genuine ailments. It does them no good when a doctor sends them away, saying, "It's all in your head. The lab tests are negative."

I welcomed these "rejects" into my practice. I took their symptoms seriously. I learned a great deal about the effects of chronic stress on the body and on the hormonal system, and about how these effects could be measured and treated.

My patients and I learned together sometimes, because there were not many available sources of information about their specific problems. I was interested in them; I wanted to apply my understanding of how the body works to their personal experiences and symptoms. Often I found illnesses that any conventional doctor could have detected, had he/she been willing to listen. Many times, too, I found that my patients had several complex problems, and that each problem affected the other.

An example of this is someone with a chronic infection (such as a parasite) who also has hypothyroidism (low thyroid hormone) and adrenal fatigue. This person would be tired and cold, gain weight and have difficulty losing it, would be slow to heal from infections, and would very likely have a poor response if given thyroid medication because of the adrenal problems. They would also complain of weakness and fatigue and disturbed digestion and diarrhea. The decrease in metabolic rate from the thyroid problem might well increase the activity of the parasitic infection too, making the gastrointestinal symptoms worse. Perhaps a gastroenterologist would figure out the parasite infection, but often these connections are missed since cultures can be negative if only one sample is done. Many endocrinologists would miss the hypothyroidism as well because standard practice calls for only a partial test of thyroid function, and few physicians will gather the complete symptoms review necessary for an accurate assessment. This means that sub-clinical hypothyroidism is routinely undiagnosed because test results are "inside the box" of what is considered the "normal" range, even though the patient has symptoms that suggest the thyroid is not functioning well.

Most physicians also overlook adrenal fatigue, because the only officially recognized medical conditions involving cortisol and adrenaline activity are Cushing's Disease (an extreme over-activity of the adrenal gland) and Addison's Disease (the adrenal gland has stopped functioning). Both are acute conditions requiring immediate medical interventions and, sometimes, hospitalization. The slower decline of adrenal function due to chronic illness or stress, while recognized and treated by many alternative health care providers, is not considered a real medical problem by the conventional medical system.

I have taken the time to describe this complex interaction of bodily systems to illustrate why I, and other alternative, integrative health care practitioners, believe so wholeheartedly in an integrated approach to treating our patients. Often I can predict by history alone who will have abnormal thyroid tests; and I am usually right. The adrenal system, which includes the hormones adrenalin, cortisol, DHEA, and aldosterone, as well as small amounts of testosterone and estrogen, has a profound impact on our well-being and reacts very strongly to stress from our physical and emotional environment. It impacts the thyroid's function, and that in turn affects adrenal function.

Traditionally, psychiatrists have diagnosed such conditions as depression, panic disorder, post-traumatic stress disorder, bipolar disorder, or psychotic disorders. Would it surprise you to know that hormonal imbalances in the thyroid, adrenals, or sex hormones could cause all of the symptoms of these conditions? Or that there are some infections that could mimic most psychiatric disorders? It is true that antidepressants are often appro-appropriately used and have saved thousands of lives, and that the new generation of anti-psychotic medications has been beneficial in making schizophrenia and other psychiatric disorders much more tolerable. I do believe, however, that these medications are overwhelmingly over-prescribed, and that many people are given anti-depressants when all they really need is to be listened to and understood as whole human beings, whose bodies affect mind and spirit. Many times, nutritional interventions, hormonal therapies, and lifestyle modifications restore these patients to full health, rather than cover up their symptoms as an anti-depressant would, so that they can tolerate their stressful lives a bit better.

My 20 years as a psychiatrist were invaluable in teaching me about the complex relationships between the body's structure and function, and as psychiatry broadened my horizons into other fields, I started to hear the sounds of a new calling. For example, I often found medical conditions that were contributing to, or even causing, my patients' psychiatric conditions. I studied, read, searched, and I found other doctors, researchers, nutritionists, and alternative medical practitioners who were learning about these relationships too, out on the fringes of conventional medicine.

I saw how profoundly hormone imbalances of many types (cortisol, adrenaline, progesterone, testosterone, insulin, estrogen, thyroid) affected mental health and general well-being. I realized that depression could make people physically and medically ill; that even lack of sleep or chronic pain could have a negative physiological impact, by, for instance, changing the hormonal balance. I found nutritional and amino acid therapies that worked better for some people than standard medications. I could see I was onto something important, but I often felt that I was struggling with these discoveries alone.

You can imagine my joy when I found out, while attending my first conference of the American Academy of Anti-Aging Medicine in 1997, that there were hundreds of practicing doctors who thought along the same lines as I did. It was like being an orphan and suddenly discovering I had a huge extended family welcoming me to a big reunion! At that time, there were only 1,200 or so attendees at the conference. Now, a decade later, this organization (which seeks to disseminate information concerning innovative science, research, and treatment modalities designed to enhance and prolong human life) has more than 20,000 members worldwide and over 5,000 health care providers attend its conferences, a good indication of the rise in popularity and acceptance of alternative methods.

I no longer feel like a lonely renegade. I still practice outside of the conventional medicine model. The difference is that now I am part of a worldwide movement, so I am no longer alone! Besides the American Academy of Anti-Aging Medicine, there are other organizations providing education and alternatives to the conventional approach to healthcare: The Life Extension Foundation, The Institute for Functional Medicine, American College of Alternative Medicine, and many, many more.

I think medicine today has become worse than mediocre in most cases. A lot of this sorry state has to do with the pharmaceutical and insurance industries' hold on doctors and patients. I alluded to this state of affairs in the Preface and will talk about it in more detail in a little while.

I do use prescription medicines when the need is urgent and a natural substance cannot help quickly enough to prevent severe injury or disability. But my goal is to prevent illness in the first place, to help the body heal itself with nutrients, diet, healthy lifestyle, information, and products that the body is familiar with and knows how to handle (rather than synthetics that have unpredictable and often dangerous effects). Every year, I am able to find more and more resources that are great stores of knowledge about human health, prevention of disease, and healing. I have also met hundreds of people who are dissatisfied with traditional medicine, but do not know how to find effective and safe alternatives. This book will help those people find the means to become informed and empowered consumers of health care.

I also see that many people are angry at the arrogant and dismissive way they are treated by doctors, insurance companies, or hospital staff. I have worked one-on-one with many patients, showing them how to be more powerful, teaching them their rights, intervening to get them information that is being withheld from them. I am angry and fed up with this system too, but I feel more optimistic than ever that things can and will change to benefit you, the individual, if only *you* are willing to act.

I am happy to share with you what I have learned. Together we can declare our independence from the many myths that bind us to a huge financial burden resulting from health care that does not make or keep us well. It is high time for change!

I am speaking to you as both a patient and a physician. I am a product of a flawed system as well. Together, we can make a meaningful and affirmative difference.

Tedde Rinker, D.O.

Chapter 2

Look Out For Number One

I have given a lot of thought to my motivations and qualifications for writing this book. The motivation is my deep concern for the health and well-being of all patients; I genuinely care about both of those aspects. With regard to qualifications, I am a licensed and Board Certified physician and surgeon, with a long list of post-graduate medical studies behind me. This certainly puts me in a position to be able to investigate, witness, and participate in the health care of thousands of people. Any physician practicing medicine today could make that claim, but most of them would not see the need for a book such as this.

My qualifications are also based on many years of practice, during which I met countless patients and cared for them as a doctor, intern, and a fortunate student of some of the best medical practitioners out there. I have heard their stories of anger, frustration, and betrayal from the mainstream medical profession. Often they come to me because I listen and help them understand what their doctor *really* said, since clear explanation of the diagnosis or treatment was sadly lacking.

I also hear horror stories of women who needlessly lost their fertility, or were given toxic medications for years, only because their doctors did not listen to them. Some people tell me their relatives died due to carelessness or the lack of attention to a symptom easily recognizable as serious.

I have taught patients that they have a right to be in charge of their health care, their charts, and their lives, and to participate in the decision making process of their treatment every step of the way. They have the right to know what I am thinking when I say that dreaded word: "hmmm."

Now I want to teach *you* about your rights as a patient, as well as the qualifications *and limitations* of health consultants. I want you to become wise and powerful consumers of health care.

This book is for people who want excellent health care, yet feel bullied or overwhelmed by standard medical practice, and feel there must be a better alternative. So many of the patients I have seen did not get healthy as a result of medical interventions. Many times, if not most of the time, their symptoms were only suppressed or controlled. Often this would make them feel temporarily and superficially better, but in fact, they were on a slow path toward chronic poor health.

I have a patient, Mary L. (not her real name), who has been told all her life that her cholesterol levels were perfect. Recently, at age 61, she came to me because she wanted to change from synthetic to bio-identical hormones. When I see a patient, I always do a cardiac risk screen first, which is more thorough than the typical lipid level. I test for inflammatory factors, and for the different *types* of LDL (Low Density Lipoprotein), instead of what the usual cholesterol test calculates: an estimate of the total LDL. Most doctors tell patients this is the "bad cholesterol." That is only partly true. There are four types of LDL. Only three of the four can contribute to damage in the artery surface or inside the wall of the artery. The last one is beneficial in that it cleanly delivers cholesterol to the body tissues where it is used as an essential building block to almost all cells of the body, but most importantly, it is critically important to the brain, the immune system, and to the formation of hormones.

The job of LDL is to deliver cholesterol to the tissues, where it is used to make cell membranes, many hormones, and a huge percentage of brain tissues, as well as to contribute significantly to white blood cells, which safeguard our defense against cancer and other diseases. All this may sound confusing, but knowing the different types of LDL is important if one is using nutrients to improve lipid levels, rather than the "statin" drugs, which lower total LDL but may not change the ratio of most damaging LDLs.

Mary, who fully expected the cardiac risk test to be a formality, found that she had advanced arteriosclerosis (abnormal thickening and hardening of the walls of arteries) and that this finding was to be a major focus of her treatment, rather than a minor stop on her way to changing to a healthier type of hormone replacement.

I told Mary that the synthetic hormone medroxyprogesterone, prescribed by her doctor and which she had been taking for two years, could very well be accelerating her arteriosclerosis, but that taking the natural progesterone would not have this effect. The acceleration of plaque formation caused by synthetic hormones was documented in the large scale Women's Health Initiative Study (WHI) of 1991, but many people do not know that there were published studies long before the WHI that concluded that synthetic progesterone cancelled out the cardiac benefits of estradiol (a natural hormone) and caused arterial vascular spasm[1].

Mary is not the only one who has been victim to this kind of uninformed, hormone-related medical care. Many of the female patients who come to me have been on oral synthetic estrogens, and I routinely find that the reason they are having so much trouble losing weight is that they are seriously estrogen dominant. They have all been put on the same dose, "one size fits all" hormone replacement, and have never had their hormone levels checked.

I wish I could say that this situation is rare, but, in fact, it is the most common problem I see in women who have been on oral synthetic hormones. It is difficult to reverse this metabolic cul-

---

[1] *Natural Hormone Balance for Women: Look Younger, Feel Stronger, and Live Life with Exuberance* (Paperback), by Uzzi Reiss; January 2, 2002; published by Atria.

Medroxyprogesterone acetate and dihydrotestosterone induce coronary hyperreactivity in intact male rhesus monkeys. [J Clin Endocrinol Metab. 2005]

J Clin Endocrinol Metab. 1998 Feb;83(2):649-59. Ovarian steroid protection against coronary artery hyperreactivity in rhesus monkeys. Minshall RD, Stanczyk FZ, Miyagawa K, Uchida B, Axthelm M, Novy M, Hermsmeyer K

J Reprod Med. 1999 Feb;44(2 Suppl):180-4.Progestogens and cardiovascular disease. A critical review. Clarkson TB.

Atherosclerosis. 2006 Dec;189(2):375-86. Epub 2006 Jan 24. Randomized trial of hormone therapy in women after coronary bypass surgery. Evidence of differential effect of hormone therapy on angiographic progression of disease in saphenous vein grafts and native coronary arteries.

Ouyang P, Tardif JC, Herrington DM, Stewart KJ, Thompson PD, Walsh MN, Bennett SK, Heldman AW, Tayback MA, Wang NY; Estrogen and Graft Atherosclerosis Research (EAGAR) Investigators.

Johns Hopkins University School of Medicine, John Hopkins Bayview Medical Center, Division of Cardiology, 4940 Eastern Avenue, Baltimore, MD 21224, USA. pouyang@jhmi.edu

de-sac, but it can be done, over several months. It is too bad that physicians do not test blood levels and do not seem to know much about hormone metabolism. And, of course, the pharmaceutical company product representatives do not encourage this kind of inquiry; they never mention hormone blood levels.

My years of practice introduced me to a multitude of patients like Mary, suffering from a variety of symptoms. Is it any wonder that I began to feel that the treatment they received was not medicine? This was not healing. I knew there was information available "out there" (which includes medical journals, basic science literature, alternative health care research, and practice) offering more than a quick fix of the presenting symptoms. Where was the motivation to go beyond the superficial?

It is a sad reality, but there are components of conventional medicine that make a profit from our illness, and they are not likely to change their structure or motives, even if they are made aware of our desire for excellence in health care. The patient is not their priority.

The message is clear: It is time to start looking out for Number One...and that's *you.* It is time to learn how to demand complete information on prevention and reversal of disease, and to learn how to analyze and use the information you have to your maximum benefit. That maximum benefit–the end result and the bottom line–should be great health. Settle for nothing less.

Chapter 3

The Law Is On Your Side

As I mentioned in the Foreword, the U.S. Advisory Commission on Consumer Protection and Quality in the Health Care Industry issued, in 1998, a "Patient Bill of Rights," with the intent to inform consumers of the rights they have with regard to medical care. I will present this below, and you will no doubt notice that these rights are not routinely extended to you when you see a health care provider. If you feel that they are, you are very fortunate indeed:

1. **Information Disclosure:** You have the right to receive accurate and easily understood information about your health plan, health care professionals, and health care facilities. If you speak another language, have a physical or mental disability, or just don't understand something, assistance will be provided so you can make informed health care decisions.

2. **Choice of Providers and Plans:** You have the right to a choice of health care providers that is sufficient to provide you with access to appropriate high-quality health care.

3. **Access to Emergency Services:** If you have severe pain, an injury, or sudden illness that convinces you that your health is in serious jeopardy, you have the right to receive screening and stabilization emergency services whenever and wherever needed, without prior authorization or financial penalty.

4. **Participation in Treatment Decisions:** You have the right to know all your treatment options and to participate in decisions about your care. Parents, guardians, family members, or other designated individuals can represent you if you cannot make your own decisions.

5. **Respect and Nondiscrimination:** You have the right to considerate, respectful, and nondiscriminatory care from your doctors, health plan representatives, and other health care providers.

6. **Confidentiality of Health Information:** You have the right to talk in confidence with health care providers and to have your health care information protected. You also have the right to review and copy your own medical record and request that your physician amend your record if it is not accurate, relevant, or complete.

7. **Complaints and Appeals:** You have the right to a fair, fast, and objective review of any complaint against your health plan, doctors, hospitals, or other health care personnel. This includes complaints about waiting times, operating hours, the conduct of health care personnel, and the adequacy of health care facilities.[2]

It is time for us to look beyond the recommendations of an advisory panel and make some declarations of our own. As long as we continue to allow the physician, the insurance provider, and

---

[2] www.consumer.gov

the big pharmaceutical companies to control our access to certain medical treatments and to a wide range of medical information, even the information about our own health, we will be bullied and intimidated by their perceived "clout." It is precisely for that reason—to inspire and guide you—that I created the Declaration of Independence for Health Care, which I included in the Foreword. Read it, memorize it, frame it if you must, but make sure it becomes your point of reference from now on.

Our Declaration of Independence for Health Care will serve as a guideline for the challenges before us. We need to free ourselves from the myths that many of us believe—often without ever voicing them aloud—that determine our behaviors when seeking and submitting to health care. Making the declaration, and taking it seriously, is the first step. Learning how we came to accept these false beliefs and unlearning them so that we can become discerning consumers of health care is the next step. The last step is finding the reliable resources to follow through to get what we need. I invite you, the reader and health care consumer, to join in this Declaration of Independence. Let's make our own standards clear to ourselves and to those who deal with us. Once we know where we stand, we can begin to march to a different drummer. The choices are many, and you are the one with the power to choose. I will help you find the resources to make those important decisions.

Chapter 4

Be A "Healthy" Skeptic

If you are lucky enough to be healthy, you want to do everything in your power to stay that way. If you are sick, you have to take every feasible and reasonable action to get well. You may not have time to let history decide which health care theories are right. Thanks to the Internet, you have the world at your fingertips and lots of help at hand.

The historical example below illustrates how many lives can be lost due to ignorance, arrogance, and lack of curiosity. After all, history really is the best teacher!

In 1794, Alexander Gordon, a Scottish surgeon, first came up with a novel (for that time) idea that doctors should wash their hands before doing vaginal examinations of pregnant women. Many women of the time were dying of puerperal fever, a life-threatening infection contracted during or shortly after childbirth, and usually caused by unsanitary conditions. Puerperal fever was rife, but physicians were insulted at the suggestion that they were causing these infections themselves, and disregarded Gordon's call for action.

In 1843 Oliver Wendell Holmes, a renowned American doctor and writer, agreed with Dr. Gordon, about the connection between unwashed hands and the spread of puerperal fever, and published a paper on the issue. Finally, Dr. Ignaz Phillip Semmelweis, a respected Hungarian physician, observed that puerperal fever was more frequent in hospitals where interns practiced on cadavers and then went on to examine pregnant women, than among women who bore children with midwives who commonly practiced hand washing. When Semmelweis later became the head of a hospital surgical unit, he performed controlled studies in which some of his operating rooms had compulsory hand sterilization in a chlorine solution prior to entry for all medical staff, while others did not have such stringent hygiene guidelines. His research clearly showed increased survival rates of mothers and infants treated by doctors who soaked their hands in a chlorinated solution.

Despite Dr. Semmelweis's ardent attempts to persuade his fellow physicians of the importance of asepsis (maintaining a sterile environment), he was ignored. At his death in 1865 (ironically, he died from an infection caused by a surgical cut to his finger), the debate about perpetuating a sterile environment in hospitals continued, but the practice was still not widely adopted.

Two decades later, a speaker in Paris expressed his skepticism about Dr Semmelwies's theory but was shouted down by Dr. Louis Pasteur, the famed French physician who had by then identified the bacteria that caused puerperal sepsis. Almost a century had passed between the time Alexander Gordon recommended hand washing and Dr. Pasteur's irrefutable proof that physicians themselves were causing transmission of this disease through lack of hygiene. How many women died unnecessarily in childbirth in those years? How many other patients underwent abdominal surgery and died for the same reason in nearly 100 years of ignorance?

During these 100 years, some women (but certainly not the majority) knew which hospitals had high death rates and which were safer—even if they did not know why—and were willing to accept extremely crowded conditions at the few hospitals practicing sanitary techniques. Often these safer hospitals were the crowded public institutions rather than the posh private ones, though they did not know that sanitizing of the hands was the critical difference.

These women were the early version of informed and discerning consumers (although they probably did not think of themselves in these terms): people who took their lives and health seriously enough to take action, without having *all* the data to draw a *scientific* conclusion themselves. They did not need a double-blind placebo crossover study to tell them that they were more likely to survive childbirth in one hospital rather than another. They had not read Semmelweis's research. Sadly, even today, when we know with certainty the dangers of passing infection from one patient to another, several observational studies done in the 1990's showed that many physicians do not wash their hands between patients.[3]

Is it always so difficult to get professional acceptance of new ideas, even ones as simple and inexpensive (and as old) as hand washing? Yes, unfortunately it is.

How can you be a powerful advocate for your own best health care in such an environment? Be a skeptic. Use whatever resources you have to find out as much as you can about all the alternatives for good health and recovery from illness. People who have the money to pay for what they want may seem to have

---

[3] Semmelweis: A Lesson in Epidemiology King-Thom Chung and Christine L. Case SIM News 47(5):234-237, 1997

an advantage, but if they are not questioning and investigating their health care, they will just get expensive treatments that have no greater chance of making them feel well than someone without money. Even for those with limited medical coverage, there are tremendous resources available to anyone who is willing to look. Do not be reluctant to question your health care providers if you are not completely comfortable with their recommendations. Trust your instincts and voice your doubts.

Chapter 5

Separating Fact From Fiction

We Americans like pills. They're promoted by their manufacturers as a quick and easy fix. It is confusing to sort through the data and read between the lines for the "spin" that the pharmaceutical and nutraceutical companies put on their products in order to seduce us into seeing their products as a "cure" for our ills.

I am a trained scientist and physician and even for me it is not easy. Sometimes these greatly heralded claims actually are cures. We certainly do have remedies for ills that people in the past would consider miraculous. But many products have undisclosed or unexplored dangers. The past and recent revelations about D.E.S, (Diethylylstilbesterol), a synthetic estrogen drug widely given to pregnant women in the 1950's through the 1970's, and thought to reduce the risk of miscarriage, is a good example. Not only did it have little impact on preventing miscarriage, it actually *increased* the risk of cancer and abnormal uterine development in the daughters born to women who took the drug.

Now it appears to have increased the cancer risk in exposed sons as well.

Other big mistakes in Pharmacology: Thalidomide, (severe disfiguring birth defects); Baychol (one of the first cholesterol reducing statin drugs to be taken off the market because of dangerous side effects and death); Vioxx (prescribed for pain and inflammation, but causing thousands of heart attacks and deaths); and many, many other recalls, far too numerous to mention here.

It is not only pharmaceutical drugs that require your scrutiny. Even "natural" supplements can have risks. Little was known about the potential bleeding problems caused by a popular herbal supplement, gingko biloba. Then some people bled to death in surgery because surgeons did not know that their patients were taking this supplement and were not aware that it could cause delayed clotting.

That does not mean ginkgo biloba is a bad supplement. It can act as an antioxidant on lipid membranes, improve memory and circulation in the brain, and reverse the sexual side effects that are commonly found with antidepressant medications.[4]

---

[4] Cohen AJ, Bartlik B.Ginkgo biloba for antidepressant-induced sexual dysfunction, J Sex Marital Ther. 1998 Apr-Jun;24(2):139-43

Boveris AD, Galleano M, Puntarulo S. In vivo supplementation with Ginkgo biloba protects membranes against lipid peroxidation. Phytother Res. 2007 Aug;21(8):735-40

Naik SR, Panda VS. Antioxidant and hepatoprotective effects of Ginkgo biloba phytosomes in carbon tetrachloride-induced liver injury in rodents. Liver Int. 2007 Apr;27(3):393-9.

Satvat E, Mallet PE.Chronic administration of a Ginkgo biloba leaf extract facilitates acquisition but not performance of a working memory task.Psychopharmacology (Berl). 2008 Jul 2.

However, you have to know that any supplement, synthetic or natural, may have risks. You have to know that there are interactions between herbal medicines and medications. No one else will be as cautious and meticulous on your behalf as you could be, if only you had the right tools. A glance at the label will seldom arm you with sufficient information to base your choices. Even some common foods, such as grapefruit juice, affect almost a hundred different medications by interfering with how the body breaks them down. That could lead to dangerously high levels of some medications in your body.

In addition to the perils of drug reactions and side effects, there are also complicating distractions faced by your health care provider. While attempting to treat you, your doctor also looks over his or her shoulder at the medical board, which expects him or her to perform within "the standard of care for the community." Because of this added pressure, your physician may be afraid to treat you any way other than what the average practitioner in the community would. And that is typically dictated by "trends" enormously influenced by—you guessed it—the pharmaceutical industry's marketing and sponsored research.

As an example, let's take the controversy over the anti-inflammatory drug Vioxx. It was removed from the market after thousands of people died from heart attacks that were finally attributed to the drug itself and not to other causes. Bextra and Celebrex, similar anti-inflammatories, were also suspected. (All three drugs were heavily promoted by their manufacturers—

(footnote 4 continued from previous page)

DeKosky ST, Furberg CD.Turning over a new leaf: Ginkgo biloba in prevention of dementia? Neurology. 2008 May 6;70(19 Pt 2):1730-1

Birks J, Grimley EV, Van Dongen M Ginkgo biloba for cognitive impairment and dementia.Cochrane Database Syst Rev. 2002;(4):CD003120 you've no doubt seen the television ads, and your doctor is visited by drug reps (salespersons) every day, promoting every conceivable brand name drug.) I received an analysis from my personal insurance carrier stating that they had reviewed their entire patient database for the past 10 years. They found that patients on Bextra and Celebrex appeared to have almost double the number of hospitalizations for cardiac procedures, and showed a significantly higher risk of cardiac death than patients prescribed Ibuprofen, Naproxen, and other, older non-steroidal anti-inflammatory drugs. Most of these "safer" drugs, as presented by the insurance companies are generic, and far less expensive. Bextra and Celebrex are still on the market, but insurers often require authorizations prior to approval of a prescription (they want the doctor to provide more info to prove that the patient really needs these drugs and cannot be treated with non-steroidal anti-inflammatory medications). Vioxx, by the way, is still fighting to get back on the market.

How can you be vigilant enough to find out about potential dangers before you are a victim of an adverse drug reaction? It is hard to make sense of it all, know your choices, and take control of your health—but you must! If you do not, you will be handing over your destiny to people who are paying more attention to pressures from the pharmaceutical and nutritional industries or insurance companies than to your health.

Though—like the majority of health care consumers—you may not have a medical education, you are stuck with the daunting job of protecting yourself from unnecessary, improper, or even downright dangerous medical treatment, as well as incomplete or inadequate evaluations. Of course, avoidance of all health care providers is not an option, because if you become ill, you need to be treated. But the old saying is true: "Knowledge is power." If you are informed about the potential pitfalls of a particular treatment and are aware of all the available options to it, and if that knowledge makes you question your health care provider, that is a good starting point. If you are also motivated to learn enough to defend yourself from being bullied out of quality health care, then you will find much assistance in these pages.

It is tempting, when faced with such an enormous task, to give up and just go to the doctor your insurance company will reimburse. You may want to take the easy and convenient road by accepting the five to ten minutes you will be allotted to state your symptoms, minimizing or even stifling your questions, be examined (or not), and receive a prescription. Some very opinionated, powerful people (doctors, insurance and drug companies, news media, the American Medical Association, and other organizations) will try to convince you that you are doing the *only* wise and practical thing.

Not so! You can and must do more for your own health. You cannot afford to depend on your health care providers for an evidence- and research-based presentation of treatment options and their risks and benefits. As a proactive consumer, using some of the tools we will later discuss in detail, you will need to arm yourself with the facts you need to properly evaluate the treatments your doctor proposes—and to recognize when your doctor's "standard of care" is not optimal, or your doctor is close-minded.

"All those other guys are quacks," is the most common dismissal I hear from traditional medical practitioners about anyone who practices outside of the standard, mainstream medical model. You know what? Sometimes they are. Oftentimes, however, these providers are the only ones really listening to you, and will actually have the right answer to your particular problem. Many of these so-called "quacks" are responsible and respected scientists who have discovered viable alternative treatments for illnesses or prevention and reversal of disease processes, but do not yet have the backing and recognition of the majority of practicing physicians. In fact, if there is no profit in these concepts, chances are the alternative practitioners may never have the whole-hearted support of any of the organizations that control the so-called "standard of care." There is a world of healing power outside of its boundaries.

Chapter 6

The Proven Wonders of Alternative Medicine

Many (if not most) traditional health care providers may not want to admit it, but studies show that complementary and alternative medicine (CAM) is growing in popularity. CAM is a group of diverse medical and health care systems, practices, and products that are not presently considered part of conventional medicine. Some health care providers practice both CAM and conventional medicine. The list of therapies that are considered complementary (used in conjunction with conventional medicine) and alternative (used in place of conventional treatments) changes continually, as some therapies are gradually incorporated into conventional health care and as other, new alternative approaches to health care emerge.

According to a nationwide government survey released in 2004, 36 percent of U.S. adults use some form of CAM. The survey was conducted as part of the Centers for Disease Control and Prevention's (CDC) 2002 National Health Interview Survey. It included questions on 27 types of CAM therapies commonly used in the United States, such as acupuncture and chiropractic, as well as therapies that do not require a provider, like natural products (herbs or botanical products), special diets, and megavitamin therapy.

Interestingly, the survey also found that about 28 percent of adults used alternative therapies because they believed conventional medical treatments would not help them with their health problem.

I was ushered into the world of CAM some years ago by my accidental discovery of Chinese medicine. Traditional Chinese medicine is a system of therapies that is considered alternative in the west, but is practiced as conventional medicine in the east. It includes a range of medical practices that originated in China and have developed over several thousand years. Traditional Chinese medicine is based on an ancient concept of balanced, vital energy flowing throughout the body. The energy is believed to regulate a person's spiritual, emotional, mental, and physical balance and be influenced by the opposing forces of yin (negative, or receptive energy) and yang (positive, or active energy).

Twenty years ago, I was traveling with a group in Mexico, and on the last day of our trip, we ate raw oysters at a fine restaurant on the coast. A month later, 15 of us were quite ill with all the signs of acute hepatitis: jaundiced, weak, constipated, and dehydrated. My lab tests showed bilirubin (part of the bile, made in the liver and stored in the gallbladder) and liver enzymes so high that the lab technician told me she had to dilute my serum three times to have the levels register on the chart!

My internist's diagnosis was that I had Acute Viral Hepatitis. He told me I should expect to be quite ill for at least two months and that there was nothing that could be done other than bed rest and drinking lots of fluids. I was so sick I could barely lift my arms.

A friend of mine brought over a young Korean doctor, whose English was not good, and the tea he made for me was even worse. He apologized and said the cure for hepatitis is the second worst tasting cure in Chinese medicine. I meant to ask him what the first one was for so I could be vaccinated against it! He also put a couple of needles in my arm and leg.

Within 20 minutes, I was able to sit up and talk with weak animation. The doctor said I should see him every day for a week or two. After what he did in 20 minutes, I was hopeful; but he also said I had to drink this awful tea four times a day! "It doesn't matter if you sweeten," he said. What he meant was, no amount of sweetening would help. Believe me, I tried. Yet, this horrible medicine was making me feel better as I gagged it down.

I saw the doctor every day for a week for acupuncture and a fresh supply of "Gag-Me" tea (my name for it). By the end of that week I was feeling much better, and after two weeks there was no sign of hepatitis. I felt great! By Chinese Medical standards, the doctor said, I was cured. He was curious to find out whether my western doctor would also declare me cured and suggested that I get re-tested for hepatitis. I did, and all my tests were back to normal or nearly normal. My friends, who had gone on the Mexico trip with me and contracted hepatitis at that same restaurant, were still severely ill.

I went to see the internist who had diagnosed the hepatitis in the first place and had told me there was no treatment other than lengthy bed rest. I was glowing with health, and bursting to tell him my story. He looked at the lab tests, examined me, and said, "Well, I guess you didn't have hepatitis after all." Shocked, I asked, "Why do you say that? There are the other people from my group who still have hepatitis!" He responded that hepatitis could not be cured so quickly. "It must have been a blocked biliary duct or something like that. Or it could be a lab error, but not hepatitis." I explained the treatment I had received for the past two weeks, but he did not budge. The physician who had diagnosed me with acute hepatitis refused to believe what was right in front of his eyes and dismissed the evidence as a laboratory error, rather than challenge and question the beliefs he had held all his life.

This was some years before the lab test for exposure to hepatitis was available. When that test later became available, I was tested for exposure to both Hepatitis A (the acute, self-limiting form of the infection which makes one quite ill for approximately two months) and Hepatitis B (chronic, often progressive, can sometimes be symptom free years later while the disease is still progressing). I tested positive for a past infection of Hepatitis A. I knew that I really had contracted hepatitis after the Mexico adventure, but even as a doctor, I still felt that I had to prove to myself that my experience was valid. It can be intimidating when a professional dismisses your symptoms and observations, even when you may be certain of them.

This personal experience of mine, dating back more than 20 years, makes me realize, from the patient's perspective, how offhandedly and ineffectively I was treated by a conventional doctor, even though I was a physician myself. If a medical colleague can do that to another physician, he/she does it even faster to a patient who is less educated in medicine. I learned something very important, but unfortunately, my internal medicine specialist, shielded by his arrogance, had not.

Chinese medicine and Western medicine operate on different paradigms.[5] They have entirely different views of how the body functions, how it is put together, why it works that way, and even how to read the signs and symptoms of the body. There are some overlapping treatments and diagnoses but, surprisingly, not as many as you might expect.

In post-revolutionary China, Chairman Mao Tse Tung ordered that both Western and Oriental medicine be studied and compared. Whichever proved to be the most effective would be the one used in China henceforth. The result of the study showed that the two systems were equally effective overall, with Chinese medicine being better in some areas, such as the treatment of viruses and chronic illnesses, and Western medicine excelling in acute conditions where emergency surgery or intravenous antibiotics are required. So, Chairman Mao allowed both in China. They exist side by side in the U.S. too, but most Americans have very little knowledge of when and how to use the services of an Oriental Medical Doctor (OMD). Most states have limited the OMD to the license of Acupuncturist, though the majority are also trained in herbal medicine.

OMD's, even if their license to practice is limited to acupuncture, attend school for several years, studying herbal medicines, clinical diagnosis, and anatomy in both the western and Oriental manner. Practitioners are guided by detailed body maps of acupuncture points, meridian lines, and anatomical sites that do not correlate with the structure of visible organs but instead with observed phenomena of the path of symptom changes through the body or temperature changes on the skin. The science and practice of physical diagnosis is also very refined in Oriental Medicine. The pulse itself is studied to a depth not explored in

---

[5] *The Web That Has No Weaver: Understanding Chinese Medicine* (Paperback) by Ted J. Kaptchuk; McGraw-Hill; 1 edition (April 11, 2000)

the Western medicine; the iris of the eye, the characteristics of the face, body, and tongue are also analyzed.

The Oriental doctor primarily uses herbs and acupuncture for treatment, but also employs some forms of massage, aromatherapy, and dietary adjustments. He/she will also recommend spiritual or emotional work that is believed to be necessary to recovery. In my case, part of my treatment recommendations for hepatitis was to learn how to express anger better. I was surprised by this assessment and was quite ready to dismiss it as irrelevant because I "knew" that my disease was caused by a virus. However, I did find it very difficult at that time to discuss angry feelings with anyone to whom I was close. I did not manage to resolve this difficulty in the two weeks that it took the Korean doctor to cure me, but I felt that it was probably worthwhile to address this issue anyway. I do not admit to understanding the relationship between anger and hepatitis, but I can certainly say that learning to resolve this difficulty has benefited me in many areas of my life.

My wish is to support you in learning about Chinese and related types of Oriental Medicine, as well as other alternative healing practices, so that you can benefit from my experience (without having to get hepatitis like I did!). With this and other knowledge you will acquire by reading this book you'll be ready to become a full partner with your health care practitioner. If you cannot persuade him or her that this kind of relationship is better for both of you, and if your arguments fall on deaf ears, find another doctor. The more insistent we become in accepting nothing less than a full partnership with our medical consultants, the better off we will be.

Chapter 7

There Are Many Roads to Good Health

This book will give you specific tools meant to prepare you to become your own health care advocate. As you continue to read, you will understand why it is so important to use these tools to better your own health, protect your rights to privacy, and redefine the relationship between you and the health care consultant. The more convinced you become that you do not have to settle for less than great health and complete communication from health care providers, the more resourceful you will become in making sure that this happens.

Knowledge of your alternatives, as they relate to health care, is an essential part of your toolbox. Both traditional, western medical approaches and complementary and alternative paths to healing should be considered in your quest for the finest health care available. In Chapter 22, we will talk specifically about how you can find the right physician or other health care provider (HCP), whether he or she is a part of the world of conventional or alternative medicine. The chapter you are reading now provides an overview of the major components of Complementary and Alternative Medicine and a structure for your research into the various non-conventional medical practices.

A search for a general definition of CAM will give you many different answers, but the simplest one is that it is a field of health care that is an alternative to traditional medicine as it is practiced in the United States and much of Europe.

Here are the most common major categories of complementary and alternative medical practice:

Acupuncture/Acupressure: This therapeutic intervention originated more than 4,000 years ago from the medical practices of the Chinese, Korean, and Indian cultures. Traditional Chinese Medicine, to which I referred earlier in the book, uses acupuncture to regulate the body's flow of Qi, or "vital energy." The insertion and manipulation of very thin needles, or the application of pressure at specific points along the meridians or channels through which Qi (or Chi) is thought to flow, is believed to correct any imbalance, excess, deficiency, or lack of fluidity in the flow of Qi.

Western culture has influenced the practice of traditional Chinese Medicine in many ways. Some long held traditions have been dropped and some newer techniques developed, but the philosophical ideas of assessment and treatment are still the same and make the Oriental medical approach different from standard western medicine for treating symptoms. The practice and techniques were developed in schools over many centuries with rigorous observation of applied techniques of diagnosis and treatment. There is a strong reliance in Chinese Medicine on observation of the body and face, the pulses, the iris of the eye, and the tongue for clues to a diagnosis. The Chinese medical practitioner also asks many questions that are not typically posed by a western physician, such as what sorts of foods are preferred, hot or cold, spicy or not, salty or bitter, etc.

Another aspect of traditional Chinese Medicine is the concept of Yin and Yang, the active and passive energies, often referred to as the female and male aspects of an action or system. These elements are all considered in the evaluation of a patient, and treatments are geared to keep the whole person in balance, to prevent disease or to restore balance. In addition to acupuncture or acupressure, massage, exercise, herbal treatments, meditation, and diet are all part of the Oriental medical intervention.

Ayurvedic Medicine: Borne out of religious scripture that dates as far back as 1200 BC, this form of CAM was considered the traditional medicine of India, although today there are more western style medical schools in India than there are Ayurvedic schools. The Ayurvedic principles of medical practice balance physical, mental, and spiritual well-being, as determined by the individual's dosha (constitution). The treatment would start with a thorough understanding of the person and his/her history, and would proceed with four important steps: Cleansing and detoxification; Reduction of negative symptoms; Rejuvenation and renewal; Mental and spiritual practices for maintenance (hygiene).

Individualized dietary plans are often recommended, based on the dosha and the season of the year. Other treatments would include herbal remedies, massage, yoga practices, and meditation and breathing exercises. I have also seen aromatherapy used in Ayurvedic treatments, as part of massage and meditation to induce certain healing states.

Homeopathy: As it is practiced in western culture today, Homoeopathy has its roots in the work of Samuel Hahnemann, a German physician who established this type of treatment about

200 years ago. The purpose is to stimulate the patient's own healing process via the administration of very small amounts of homeopathic remedies, substances that can produce in a healthy person the same symptoms as those experienced by the patient. A direct translation from the Greek, homeopathy means "same as the pathology." The homeopathic doctor conducts a detailed interview with the patient, eliciting details of the symptoms of the condition to be treated, and then prescribes in extraordinarily minute doses substances which could cause similar symptoms if given in a larger dose. The concept here is to use these micro dosages of a "like" compound to stimulate the response of the body to create its own antidote or healthy response to the negative symptom.

There have been other remedies developed in Homeopathy that do not have this "same as the pathogen" origin, but still utilize small dosages of substances that should do no harm. In fact, while there is no FDA input into the development of new homeopathic remedies, the institution that regulates new homeopathic compounds has three criteria which must be proven by clinical trials before a new remedy is accepted: The substance must be of very small ("micro") quantity; it must not cause any side effects greater than placebo in a comparison study; and it must show satisfactory clinical response for the condition it proposes to treat.

Chiropractic: The technique of spinal adjustment originated in ancient Egypt, where practitioners adjusted the spines of their patients to maintain health. The term Chiropractic came into use much later, in the 1800's in the United States. Today, Chiropractic medicine is based on the concept that the alignment and proper functioning of the spinal column is necessary for optimal health. Manipulation of the spine can resolve many uncomfortable and painful conditions of the neck, head, spine, arms, and legs, without the need for the pain medications or muscle relaxants typically used by Western medical doctors to treat muscle spasm and bodily pain. Many Chiropractic physicians receive or seek additional training in nutrition and will recommend nutritional supplements and herbs as part of their treatment. They are not licensed to write prescriptions for medications, but can order diagnostic X-ray studies and lab tests, and also employ other forms of physical therapy, besides manipulation, such as ultrasound and heat treatments.

Dietary and Nutritional Therapies: These are fundamental therapeutic interventions in some alternative and complementary medical practices and have been used as an essential part of treatment for thousands of years. In Traditional western medicine, dietary recommendations are also made, but are often not specific and not administered by the physician.

Non-Western cultural traditions make little distinction between food and medicine, and practitioners will prescribe specific types of food to cleanse the system or help rid the body of toxins. In Ayurvedic Medicine, certain types of spices and food temperatures are recommended based on body type. The avoidance of certain types of food is often recommended in both traditional and complementary practices for people with certain disorders. For example, with cardiac disease, it is common to recommend a reduction in animal fats and salty foods, and with diabetes, the recommendation is careful monitoring of dietary intake of food that can easily be converted to sugar, such as sweets, fruits, and starches.

Alternative and complementary practices that utilize nutritional interventions include macrobiotics, orthomolecular medicine, and various forms of vegetarianism. Macrobiotics, based on Asian concepts of nutrition, emphasizes the consumption of locally grown fruits, grains, legumes, and vegetables eaten in the proper season.

Vegetarian dietary interventions vary widely: some exclude all animal products (vegan), while others include milk and/or eggs (lacto-ovo) in the diet and/or fish. While vegetarianism is not necessarily a medical therapy per se, many practitioners may recommend certain types of vegetarian diets for a specific health reason.

A nutritional counselor may be a registered dietician or a clinical nutritionist, or may be someone who has learned a great deal about food and diet and acts in an advisory role without specific training in nutritional interventions. Some practitioners will analyze the patients' diets by having them keep a food intake journal, yet others will do clinical testing of blood, saliva, feces, and urine to help determine nutritional deficiencies, food allergies, or problems with absorption of nutrients or elimination of waste. There are many conditions with all the symptoms of a serious chronic disease that are, in fact, no more than food allergies or intolerances. I have worked with many patients who report a resolution of multiple symptoms, such as migraine headaches, joint pain, chronic abdominal pain, and fatigue, simply by eliminating foods that were causing allergic reactions.

In the field of nutrition, some health care practitioners, both alternative and mainstream, may advise people on matters of health that lie outside of their field of expertise. It is important when this happens that you find out if the HCP in question has had specific training in nutrition, and if so, what kind? For example, there are nutritionists whose training is primarily in meal planning for institutions, yet they might set up a practice and prescribe nutritional therapies with supplements and high dose vitamins, when they have not been specifically trained to do so.

Likewise, physicians are not taught much, if any, nutritional medicine in the normal course of medical school, so if they are recommending that you take, or not take, some nutrient, it would be wise to ask about their knowledge of Nutraceutical therapy. I know of many physicians who advise against nutritional supplements, believing the pharmaceutical industry's "propaganda" that opposes vitamin and mineral supplementation, without having done any medical literature searches themselves to back up their position. Keep an open mind, however, as many nutritionists and physicians can and do seek training beyond the basics of their specialties; do not dismiss their advice out of hand simply because it is not compatible with their licenses.

Massage Therapy: An intervention that is an essential part of some CAM practices, especially Oriental and Ayurvedic Medicine. It is also a modality used in physical therapy in traditional western medicine.

Generally, massage can be defined as rubbing, stroking, or applying pressure to the skin, muscles, tendons, and fascia (connective tissue) of the body for the purpose of improving circulation, mobilizing toxins, relaxing the body, and reducing pain and stress. Massage treatments are described in ancient Chinese, Egyptian, and Roman writings, and may date back before the written word. The technique was not specifically called "massage" until the late 1800's, when Per Henrik Ling, a Swedish gymnast, formulated the principles of what is now commonly known as a Swedish massage.

There are literally dozens of massage therapies that can vary from country to country and that have their own disciplinary schools and specialists. In the United States, most therapists will be experienced in more than one form of massage, and adapt the technique to the needs of the recipient. Massage therapies have been shown in clinical studies to be helpful in the treatment of anxiety, chronic pain, depression, insomnia, headaches, and back pain. They are often employed in the treatment of repetitive stress injuries and sports injuries.

Mind-Body Approaches: Mind-body medicine focuses on the interactions between the brain (mind) and the body and on the effects that emotional, mental, social, spiritual, and behavioral factors have on health. The term "mind-body" is used to describe practices that are taught as disciplines to improve physical performance and well-being and aid in relaxing and calming a stressful mind and body. Mind-body therapies can include physical stretching and movement techniques like Yoga and Tai Chi, or Qi Gong. It can also include passive/receptive techniques like guided imagery, meditation, relaxation, or hypnosis, and interactive techniques like biofeedback.

Yoga and Tai Chi, both ancient forms of meditation/exercise, began hundreds of years ago, in India and China, respectively. Yoga is focused on held positions of stretched and toned muscles accompanied by a calm and relaxed attitude that is enhanced by specific breathing techniques. Tai Chi is characterized by slow, smooth movements in a ritualized practiced pattern or "dance," and has a strong mental component as well. It can be likened to "active meditation." Studies done on Tai Chi in older adults showed that it improved mental alertness, balance, self-control, as well as bone density and muscle strength.

Western Herbalism: Western herbalism is a form of alternative medicine that emphasizes the study and use of European and Native American herbs in the treatment and prevention of illness. It is based on both clinical experience and traditional knowledge of medicinal plant remedies that have their roots in ancient times. In fact, a large number of modern pharmaceutical drugs have their beginnings in research on natural remedies, which led to the development of synthetic analogues were stronger or had a longer duration of action in the body. Some of these drugs are actually not as effective as the original herbal treatment, but as a synthetic "copy" can be patented and sold as an expensive pharmaceutical drug. One example of this is Artemisinin, an extract from the wormwood tree, which is approved by the World Health Organization as an effective treatment for malaria.

As the various types of CAM grow in popularity, botanical products as healing compounds are coming back into widespread use. Western herbalism classifies many herbs according to their opposing activity: for example, herbs may have anti-inflammatory, antimicrobial, antispasmodic, or hypotensive (blood pressure reducing) effects. Other terms describe a supportive action: for example, adaptogenic herbs (those that increase resilience and improve the stress response) and tonics (improving energy or function).

Herbal preparations may be prescribed for ingestion as teas, as capsules or tablets, or as extracts or tinctures (highly concentrated liquids). Herbs may also be prepared as an essential oil and used topically, as a balm or a salve.

Parris Kidd, PhD, is a cell biologist who lectures nationally about natural remedies for improved mental function. He also does research to document the effectiveness of natural supplements for a variety of health issues. Kidd is a strong advocate for natural medicine, but also believes that standard medical care can be equally good. “I strongly feel that there is little relationship between where a person goes to school and how they turn out as a physician (or scientist),” he says. “The real correlation is with the individual’s personal values/ethics and their educational preparation in college. An alternative school may or may not be strong on the necessary training, any more than a mainstream school is strong on imbuing good values and ethics. I believe the overall quality of the experience has to do with the matching of the patient’s combinations of expectations and values with those of the physician. Sometimes people expect that their health insurance should cover the ‘alternative’ practitioner (this term I oppose, by the way). When they have to pay out of their pockets, that can lead to a negative reaction to the entire experience."

Dr. Kidd believes that natural supplements have a powerful impact on health and well-being, but thinks that often we expect instant relief from a single pill. "There are no fast cures, either via the mainstream or the alternative movement. This seems to be the hardest thing for lay people to understand. To be healthy and stay healthy we have to work on it mindfully every day. This also applies to dietary supplementation."

Alternative health care providers, who have training beyond that of a conventional physician, are a rich source of information and healing. Naturopathic Doctors (ND's), for example, are taught the pharmacological effects of plants from around the world and how to compound tinctures, capsules, and creams from these botanicals. They can act as both a natural herbal physician and a pharmacist as well.

Traditional medical schools do not offer the training given to the Naturopath, nor to other types of alternative medical practitioner. For example, there are many occasions where one would get better treatment in the hands of a skilled Chiropractor, Podiatrist, Osteopathic physician, or a "bodyworker" (someone trained in any discipline of massage therapy) than by an Orthopedic surgeon. There are also times when your condition could worsen because you did not get proper evaluation by an orthopedic surgeon to determine if your bones or tendons could hold up to a manipulation. The dance of the specialists is one I hope to teach you before you are finished with this book.

Practitioners from both traditional and alternative medicine should be considered as potential members of your health care team. Do not think that one field excludes the other or that one is "better" than the other. Alternative or conventional, complementary or traditional – all have their place and are best used for different aspects of health care. They are all a part of a system of holistic care that considers all aspects of the patient and his or her health. Your loyalty should not lie with any particular practitioner or specialty. Your bottom line is this: which therapy provides you the most beneficial results?

Chapter 8

The Empowered Patient

In this chapter, we will examine the new phenomenon of strong, well-reasoned patients who become their own health care advocates. These patients have a high degree of intelligent skepticism of the general standard of care of western medicine. We will also discuss alternative treatments that are supported with anecdotal information: testimonials from dozens (or hundreds, and at times, even thousands) of people who have assumed control of their health, who have found a new life and a relief they never had from the traditional medical treatments. Should these treatments be considered valid if they lack verification from conventional medical research?

Here is one such testimonial from a patient I know. Scott Forsgren is a 35-year-old manager at a Silicon Valley company. He had always been health conscious, even before he became ill 10 years ago with a mysterious ailment. He experienced strange flu-like symptoms. As he remembers it, “I kept getting a really intense burning sensation throughout my entire body. I immediately started going to doctors, because I just knew this was something serious and different. I mean, I was having heart palpitations, night sweats, and things that just didn't feel like a fever. Most doctors told me it was probably some virus but that they couldn't make sense of my symptoms, so I started going from doctor to doctor, with no results. At that point, I was even having trouble getting up and walking across the room. I was probably in bed 16 hours a day."

Scott's daily routine focused on struggling through his workday, often going to the bathroom to vomit, and feeling as if he were moving through a fog. These mystifying symptoms continued, and Scott remembers that for about nine months he visited doctor after doctor trying to find an answer. He was told he might have Multiple Sclerosis and had a CAT scan and an MRI of his brain, but these tests did not confirm the diagnosis. Another specialist thought he had food allergies, and evaluations for that did not solve the mystery either.

Finally, one physician tested Scott for intestinal parasites, and that result came back positive. He had also been diagnosed with Chronic Fatigue Syndrome. With those possible diagnoses, Scott looked for the best expert he could find. "I found a doctor who was practicing in Arizona, an expert in the field who had written a book on chronic fatigue syndrome, and I flew out there and met with him. He looked at the parasitic results and the overall symptoms and concluded that I should be treated aggressively with a lot of drugs. Unfortunately, my symptoms didn't really go away. I was still having a lot of neurological stuff–muscle twitches, burning sensations in my skin, etc."

Scott spent two years working with this doctor, and was on several regimens of drugs that should have cured his intestinal parasites. By the year 2000, Scott reported that he felt almost back to normal. Later he would find out that, coincidentally, many of the drugs used for parasites also are used to treat Lyme disease, a factor that would come into play four years later.

However, at that point Scott felt much better and stopped taking antibiotics. He attributed his remaining symptoms to having been exposed for a long time to strong medications.

By 2002, Scott believed he was well but continued to experience some unexplained symptoms. "I began having a lot of visual disturbances, so I started going to eye surgeons and saying, 'What's going on?' They couldn't find anything. I also had a couple of other symptoms, such as weird tastes in my mouth for weeks at a time. So, I went to doctors and was tested for all the parasites again, but nothing ever showed up. Most of the time the symptoms disappeared by themselves. I knew there were some residual issues and damage that I thought was related to my immune system being 'whacked out' for so long."

In September of 2004, all of the neurological symptoms, including the burning sensations, returned. "I felt like someone had poured acid all over my body or that I had stayed out in the sun for eight hours, even though you couldn't see anything on my skin," Scott says. "I also had numbness and tingling and I couldn't feel my arms or legs when I was sleeping. I found another doctor in Napa, CA, who treats parasites. At this point, we didn't consider that maybe there was something other than parasites causing my problems. That came later."

In his quest for healing, Scott visited yet another practitioner, one who treats parasitic infections, as well as disorders like Lyme disease and other problems, and uses both conventional and alternative treatments. Even though Scott presented many of the specific symptoms (blurred vision, light sensitivity, muscle spasms, tingling and burning, digestive issues, fevers and night sweats, and heart palpitations) that are seen in Lyme disease, the doctor never suggested this tick-borne illness as a cause. "He did suggest that I go to this little clinic where a woman uses a computer and does electrodermal screening [a technique using a computerized instrument to evaluate health by detecting energy imbalances along the acupuncture meridians identified in Chinese medicine]. Though this method may not be considered scientific by conventional medicine, the woman told me I had Lyme disease. She was using a BioSET™ device through the computer, introducing the frequencies of these infections and seeing if my body produced a stress response or not. I looked around this scene and thought, 'I'm at an outlet mall, next to a Starbucks, talking to a lady who thinks I have this horrible disease—what a nutcase!'"

To make a long story short, that woman was right—Scott did have Lyme disease. He went back to the doctor who had referred him to this practitioner, and requested a test for Lyme disease. The test was positive. All of the symptoms he had been suffering all these years were now explained by the new diagnosis—one obtained by an obscure alternative medicine practitioner in a strip mall. "I then switched to a doctor who specialized exclusively in treating Lyme disease, and with treatment, started to improve."

Scott is back to functioning at almost full speed again, but is still battling his illness and has started a website about Lyme disease (www.betterhealthguy.com) in order to encourage discussion about the condition and to learn how other people deal with it. He also started attending medical conferences on Lyme disease and interviewing specialists for a citizen newspaper on Lyme and associated diseases called Public Health Alert. Scott is undoubtedly a model for all of us.

"I think most people, unless their condition is severely impacting their lives, will just accept whatever they are told," he notes. "But I walked out of the doc's office where I was told there's nothing wrong with me when I knew there certainly was, and I told myself, 'I'm going to keep looking for answers.' The path I'm going down right now might be completely wrong for everyone else, but I know I am functional because I kept looking for and found the pieces of the puzzle that had eluded most doctors."

Scott's experience is an example of what is called "anecdotal evidence." Anecdotal evidence is an informal report in the form of a personal testimony. It ranges from a friend telling you about a particular therapy or supplement that "worked for me" to the cultural wisdom of a non-Western society that has for centuries been using local remedies to heal disease. The term is often used in distinct contrast to the formal "scientific" evidence relied on in conventional medicine.

My own relating, in a previous chapter, of personal and observational data about the successful and effective treatment I received for hepatitis is another example of anecdotal evidence. If I were the only person in the world who ever had this experience, then the anecdote would be of little value. However, you can go to various search engines and find out if research has been done on herbal and acupuncture treatments for acute hepatitis. This is one way that you can determine if anecdotal evidence is worth considering in your quest for medical knowledge. I will help you learn how to evaluate anecdotal information in order to determine its real value. We also need to learn as much as we can about the "untold" side effects of treatments that are "proven" by evidence-based medicine.

Does the fact that knowledge of a therapy that has not been scrutinized with modern statistical techniques mean it has no value? Should you only use traditional medicine that is supported by the one specific kind of scientific data currently favored in this country because it is most useful in promoting pharmaceutical interests, or is this limiting your access to important cures and prevention? Is there legitimacy in other types of corroboration that support the value of a medical treatment? Are anecdotal reports, for instance, worth listening to? When a new treatment offers only testimonials as support for its value, does that mean the cure is only hype? How about basic science research on human physiology? There is new research being pub-published all the time that has nothing to do with marketing a new drug, but which provides a better and deeper understanding of how our bodies work and what we need to function well. These findings are published in scientific journals, biology reviews, and nutritional science journals. Right now, and in the past several years, the phrase 'evidence-based medicine" has become quite popular in health care and in the advertising of pharmaceutical products. But, what exactly does this mean?

Prior to World War II, medical dictates were established when a panel of experts would render opinions on the worthiness or effectiveness of a new treatment modality. After the war, with the advent of a large number of new pharmaceutical drugs and vaccines, there was a shift toward more reliance on an "objective" analysis of treatments (most of which were medications or vaccines). Greater objectivity was found in doing controlled studies, in which a control group received a placebo (an inactive compound) and a study group received the active substance being investigated. Neither the participants (patients) nor the observers (researchers) would know who got a placebo and who got the active substance until after all the data was gathered. This is the basic format of the "double-blind placebo-controlled study." It was very useful and effective for pharmaceutical companies attempting to assess side effects and to prove that their new drug was effective for the condition it was intended to treat. It also came to be a requirement the Food and Drug Administration placed on drug companies, to get approval to market a patented medication to the general public, and to physicians.

Since WWII, the double-blind placebo-controlled study has attained such power as a validating tool that many health professionals would not consider any treatment that had not been subjected to such a study. One of the drawbacks, however, is that participants cannot be under any other treatment or medications so as not to affect the integrity of the study's outcome. Participants are also excluded if they have more than one illness. Since there are many other exclusion factors as well, double-blind placebo-controlled studies are left with a group of volunteers who might not be much like the "average person" who would be the end user of the drug or treatment in question. Such studies are scientific, in the sense that rigorous controls are in place to obtain specific information, but what happened to clinical experience? Why is it not considered valid any more as a significant contributing factor to choosing the best treatment for the patient? There is also the patient's history.... perhaps it is different (it often is, in some way) from the patients in the controlled study? And what about environmental factors, such as diet, exposure to pollutants and toxins, and the genetic specificity of the individual? What about stress? Chronic stress or trauma can have a profound effect on health, as has been documented hundreds of times in medical literature, and is often overlooked in the assessment and treatment of a person.

As health care practitioners, we can and should evaluate *all* these variables. We certainly must not ignore research on new drugs, but we should not be swayed from observing the patients in their own environments, or from listening to what the patient wants. If the patients do not say outright what they want, then health care professionals should ask them. Patients and health care professionals have their own set of responsibilities. The health care provider's responsibility is to inform the patient of all the available treatment options, whether or not the provider offers them or even believes in them. If all of the choices are made clear, then an effective and satisfactory treatment is much more likely.

Press your doctor not only for a listing of alternative therapies, but also for details of each proposed treatment, test, or procedure: why is the treatment or test necessary; is it an outpatient procedure or will it require hospitalization; what possible ill effects might occur and how long do these effects last; does your doctor have much experience with the treatment or procedure and what is the typical outcome; how long will it take to get back the results and exactly what will these show? Inquire specifically about proposed medications/drugs: are there any natural alternatives to this drug; what are the side effects and possible adverse reactions, both short and long term; are there interactions with other drugs or with foods or supplements; how long will the medication take to work and how will you know if it's working; how long will you have to take this medication? The patient's responsibility is to ask questions and demand answers. A good doctor or other health care provider will not be offended by questions; he/she will appreciate knowing that you, the patient, are well informed and well prepared to follow through on an agreed course of treatment.

Being an informed patient and a proactive consumer of health care means that you have a full understanding of all of the variables that will enter into your decision-making processes, whether you are seeking to maintain your health or to find solutions to your health problems. If you partner with your health care provider, you will be more invested in actively pursuing the best outcome.

Chapter 9

It Is Not Always The Doctor's Fault

Health care providers operate under an unreasonable burden of infallibility, which, as modern medicine becomes more complex and alternative care becomes more accessible, should be shared equally between the medical consultant and the patient. This does require learning some humility on the part of the health care practitioner and the taking on of responsibility by the patient, but this equal partnership benefits all the parties.

I have opinions, too, that I will present openly: *a good health care practitioner <u>must</u> have the patient as an informed partner in his / her diagnosis and treatment.* I want as many people as possible—patients and health care professionals—to have access to the lessons I have learned from my patients. They have taught me that the books and double-blind studies don't have all the information there is to know about the human body and mind. A doctor and a patient should operate—no pun intended—as a team.

Medical school taught me so much. This information is vital, and I must go back and review it at regular intervals, especially physiology, biochemistry, and cellular biology. These subjects are much more useful to me today than I ever dreamed they would be when I studied them in medical school. Unfortunately, most other physicians have forgotten these subjects and have no wish to revisit them. If they did, they would be a LOT more suspicious of pharmaceutical claims.

I have learned that the way we look at the structure and function of the body and at the cure for any given disease is just <u>one</u> way to see it. I know that there are many physicians who allow conventional medical practices and their insurance companies to dictate to them how to treat patients. There are also a fair number of physicians who question the "standard of care" when it appears to change with each new pharmaceutical drug introduced onto the market, or when older drugs become available as generics. The insurance providers want to dictate the "standard" based on the least costly treatment, while the pharmaceutical companies want to drive the standard by their newest treatment, regardless of the cost, safety, or availability of equally effective alternatives. Both the health insurance providers and the pharmaceutical companies are determining the standard of care, and the bottom line is profits. The traditional doctor is in the middle and tries to please them both.

Many physicians are afraid to take on these corporate giants and to defy them, even when they know there is something seriously wrong with this system. Instead, they shortchange the patient. They shorten the visit and spend less time listening to the patient and explaining diagnosis and treatment. But we shortchange ourselves, too. Patients believe that because they pay health insurance premiums, they should not have to pay any more for health care, beyond a nominal co-payment. This is one of the issues that frightens physicians into being less than they could or want to be. I have attended many conferences on practice management, where I frequently meet physicians who bemoan the loss of control of their practice and describe the feeling that they are "owned" by insurance companies. Even if these doctors offer a good quality of care, they believe that patients will leave their practices if they defy the insurance companies and cancel their suffocating contracts. They fear that their patients will just go to the next doctor on the list who will accept their health plan.

Patients, on the other hand, are left feeling as if they are wading through a herd of uncaring and inconsiderate doctors in order to find just one who will not only listen, but also do whatever is necessary to determine the cause of their symptoms and to offer an effective treatment. Many doctors wish that they had the freedom to offer their patients what they need, but feel they cannot because they are sinking into debt and are overwhelmed by the bureaucratic and organizational pressure to "comply." If only they knew how much more valued their medical advice would be if it contained more than the memorized "standard of care" that is handed to them by the pharmaceutical and health insurance companies. The only way they will know this is if we, doctors and patients, band together, demand exactly what we want, and not settle for less.

I cannot promise you that your doctor is one of those who are eager to courageously step out of the confines imposed on them and are not afraid to stand up to the insurance and pharmaceutical industry. My guess—based on my own experience and observation—is that too many health care professionals are frightened to take that risk. However, as the song goes, "times they are a-changing." Consumers are becoming savvier and more demanding.

And that is a very good thing.

My advice is simple, though it takes learning and courage to implement. We have all been brainwashed by advertising and marketing to expect unrealistic things. Doctors are not gods, and obeying them indiscriminately will not make you thrive. Find—through referrals or people you know and trust—caring physicians and healers who understand that the insurance and pharmaceutical companies are not in this business to make sure that we, the consumers, are healthy or to make sure everyone gets the best quality care at a reasonable price. They are in this for profit, and they do not particularly care whether you survive and thrive (despite their claims to the contrary), as long as their shareholders are happy.

Health insurance companies are more like bookies at the racetrack. They take odds on the likelihood of your not demanding payment for medical care so that they can keep as much of your insurance premium as possible. That is their primary means for making a profit. They can also cut costs at the other end by pressuring providers into accepting less and less, even though the cost of providing the service (employee wages, rent, equipment, office supplies) have all gone up. The reimbursement rates to physicians have gone down in many instances. Insurance companies do make a profit. Hospitals and physician offices, on the other hand, are barely scraping by. If we expect to get high quality health care paid for 100 percent by our insurance policy, then we should perhaps move to another country.

We have the most expensive health care in the world, yet we have nowhere near the healthiest population or the best longevity rates. Do not take my word for it; check out the World Health Organization figures and you will see that, when it comes to life expectancy, the U.S. is below most of the European Union countries. We take more prescription medications in the U.S. than anywhere else in the world. Why are we not feeling great? After all, the pharmaceutical industry keeps promoting all those "miracle" drugs! Drug companies spend millions researching new products, and when they find and patent a new drug, they spend a few more millions to go through the three required stages of clinical trials to get the Food and Drug Administration (FDA) approval. They want to get this investment back plus a handsome profit.

The FDA requires that clinical trials in humans last only one year. If the pharmaceutical company has information that does not look safe or effective for the drug after two, three, or 10 years of use, they are *not required* to report it. That is a win-win situation for the drug manufacturers, wouldn't you say?

Let's consider the 1991 Women's Health Initiative Study (WHIS), a large-scale clinical trial of synthetic estrogen and progestin. The study involved 161,808 postmenopausal women and demonstrated that long-term use of these hormones may increase the risk of heart attack, strokes, blood clots, and breast cancer. Wyeth-Ayerst, the pharmaceutical giant that provided the drugs and the placebo for the research, suffered a significant decline in sales of their synthetic hormones Premarin™ and Prempro™ following the study.

Years of prior research on the naturally occurring hormones estradiol, estrone, estriol, and progesterone had shown the health benefits of hormone therapy, but Wyeth-Ayerst was not required to mention that the drugs used in the WHIS study were not the same as the ones our body produces. The research panel simply indicted *all* hormones, misleading medical associations, physicians, and consumers for years about what was safe and what was not.

In order to recoup some of its lost sales, Wyeth-Ayerst has even filed a citizen's petition to the FDA to attempt to stop women and physicians from turning to bio-identical hormones , individually compounded and based on each woman's unique needs. Bio-identical compounds have the same chemical and molecular structure as those produced by your own body, but they cannot be patented, as can synthetic hormones. This trend in prescribing bio-identical hormones has become popular enough to cut substantially into the profits of Wyeth-Ayerst. The drug company's petition claims that these hormones are unsafe and unlawful. Yet, they still promote Premarin and Prempro as the best possible choice for menopausal hormone replacement.[1]

On January 9, 2008, the FDA issued an announcement warning seven compounding pharmacies to stop putting bio-identical Estriol in compounded prescriptions for post-menopausal women, even though they were doing so at the direction of licensed physicians. Bio-identical Estriol is identical to the estriol found in women, in the highest amounts during pregnancy, and can be derived from plant products such as yam and soy.

The same announcement said that physicians and pharmacies should stop using the term "bio-identical," as it is not "scientific." This injunction is clearly directed at doctors who practice hormone therapies with the idea of matching the hormone prescription to the individual woman's physiology and ability to metabolize estrogen. There is widespread protest from patients receiving these prescriptions, and from the doctors who prescribe them. What will happen to the rights of people to get individualized prescriptions designed specifically for them is yet to be seen.

You be the judge: Is the patient's health and safety the drug companies' highest priority? The message, about the risk and

---

[1] I wonder why Wyeth Ayerst was even allowed to produce Prempro after a 1996 article published in the medical journal "Circulation" showed, in a double-blind, placebo-controlled study that adding the Provera to Premarin actually cancelled out any cardiac benefit estradiol offered and caused worsening of cardiac condition. They didn't even need the WHI to find this out!

benefit of hormone replacement therapy, from the American Medical Association and the American Academy of Obstetrics and Gynecology changes every few months to every year. With all those mixed signals, docs do not see a clear direction. And if the medical professionals have no clue which drugs are safe and effective, good luck to the rest of us!

A true scientific approach to medical care has to include attention to more than a double-blind placebo-controlled study. What about the other paths leading us to health? Those that allow for the patient's uniqueness and for the possible interactions of the environment with the body?

An intelligent, intuitive, and well-read physician who is able to take the time to consult with a patient (rather than talking at him), and take the appropriate amount of time needed to do justice to the individual concerns, is the best ally a patient could have. We can only hope that this treasure of a health care provider will not go bankrupt in the attempt to offer this most valuable service. The insurance company may not want to pay for it, and the pharmaceutical company may not like the results either. That physician will have become an alternative health care provider, a renegade.

Non-western and non-traditional paths toward achieving and maintaining good health are commonly grouped together as "alternative medicine," or, as I mentioned before, "Complimentary and Alternative Medicine" (CAM). Practitioners of CAM have a wide variety of backgrounds, and can offer many options that are not considered part of the traditional standard of care, which, as I have said, is focused on prescription medications that have been proven in a double-blind study to be effective at controlling a specific symptom or symptoms of a specific disease.

If we look at these symptoms or conditions in an entirely different way, we can come up with a different diagnosis, treatment, and cure. Some of these cures are as good as or even better than those espoused by the western medical approach.

Western medical doctors must learn to think of alternative medicine practitioners as valuable allies in the ultimate goal of finding a path toward better health for each individual. Think of it this way: Suppose that you have always believed that there was just one road to the neighboring town and you had always taken that road. Then you were told that some of your friends take a different road and get to town quicker. You might want to try that road as well. You might even discover that you like it much more than the other one.

I told you earlier in the book about my own experience with Chinese medicine, and how it proved to be far superior to the type of treatment offered by a conventional doctor for my infection with hepatitis. This personal experience shows that traditional medicine does not always have the answer for every ailment. There are many roads to good health.

The most important bottom line to both physicians and patients is this: We are all manipulated by huge industrial, medical, and pharmaceutical complexes. These businesses do not care if physicians are restricted from performing a truly thorough evaluation of a patient's symptoms or from offering their patients a range of treatment options that might lie outside of the mandated standard of care. They do not care if patients suffer severe toxic side effects from a new drug (well, it *was* listed as a possible side effect), or whether doctors are bullied into prescribing it. The "system" has a vested interest in blocking your (and your doctor's) path to complete knowledge about treatments and therapies. We all, medical professionals and health care consumers alike, have to wake up and stop letting their propaganda confuse us.

Chapter 10

An Rx For Doctors

There is a war going on. In this war, the health care practitioners and the patients are the bystanders, the pawns, and the objects on the playing fields. We are not going to be the winners. Who is fighting this war? The answer: governments, the food industry, the pharmaceutical industry, the nutraceutical industry, and the insurance industry, including offshoots such as malpractice, health, and life insurance.

Perhaps there are *some people* in these organizations who are genuinely interested in better health care for real people, but by and large, these entities are primarily interested in profit for their shareholders and lower cost to the organization. The advice I give in this book is an effort to make people aware of this agenda, and to get and deliver quality health care in spite of this reality. I do not mean to imply that these organizations are inherently evil. They can, however, put the health care provider in an impossible squeeze for time and for financial and professional survival. The “powers that be” do this by imposing those "standards of care" we have talked about, which can pressure physicians to prescribe certain medications against his/her better judgment. The implication that one medication type or treatment protocol is the “standard of care” for a certain condition implies that the treating practitioner is taking a risk in using another type of treatment, or in exploring new treatments, or sometimes by referring the patient to an alternative provider, even if this exploration is initiated and requested by the patient.

Government and industry also force health care providers to choose quantity over quality, by pressuring them to emphasize efficiency in order to survive in a small business environment. This is especially true for practitioners who accept Medicare or Medicaid, or who have contracted relationships with health insurance companies and must accept the pre-determined fee, no matter how much time they spend with a patient. Doctors do not get any training in running a small business, unless they seek it on their own. Many doctors and other health care providers come out of medical training, set up their practices, and are ruined in the first 10 years.

We did not become physicians, chiropractors, naturopaths, OMDs[2], nutritionists, homeopaths, nurse practitioners, and physician assistants to run a business, or go bankrupt trying to keep our heads above water. We were thinking about something worthwhile to do with that miraculous science of healing, the connection with human beings, and the joy of making them well. Yes, we wanted to be comfortable, appreciated, and respected for our work. We did not want patients looking for a way to take us to court, or to spend endless hours managing our books and trying to reduce the cost of overhead in our offices.

---

[2] Oriental Medical Doctor; in some states they are not allowed to use this title, despite their training, and are licensed only as Acupuncturists.

We also did not want to be forced to look at a patient as just another "case." How did we lose the ability to see patients as individuals rather than merely diseases? If you are a health care practitioner and you feel you have not lost that ability, then put this book in your waiting room. If, on the other hand, you have distanced yourself from that crucial approach to patient care, and want it back, pay attention to this book. First, read it from a patient's point of view, and then from a health care provider's. You may one day find yourself in the hands of unknown health care providers who treat you as they see fit, without your input and without your complete understanding of your diagnosis and possible alternative treatments–if you have not been in this position already.

Empowered patients are not a threat. At first they may seem so—they will demand a copy of your notes and lab reports and will want to know what your treatment plan is, as well as your differential diagnosis. They will do their homework. They will point out new findings you might not have had the time to research. They will participate in their treatment plans, and in building their charts. But with smart patients like these, medicine might be fun again.

The hard part will be that you will have to do more than simply swallow the propaganda that the pharmaceutical reps feed you. You will have to research the information yourself. But don't worry; there are resources, lots of them. It is not that pharmaceutical reps are not telling you the truth. It is just that "truth" has the rep's spin on it, and you need to know *all* the facts to make a rational decision about the best treatment for your patient, *with your patient.* It is only fair. You, as a health care professional, may want to rethink some of your provider contracts, and reconsider where you should go for continuing medical education. You could choose conferences that do not have corporate sponsors. You will be surprised at the differences in the information presented, sometimes even by the same presenter who speaks at a sponsored event.

Consider your contracts with insurance providers. Ask yourself:

1. Do they prevent you from offering the patient all the alternatives you know about, even if you do not practice them yourself?

2. Do they force you to prescribe a limited range of medications or treatments, when others would be safer or more effective?

3. Do they limit the time you can spend with a patient, so that you cannot do a complete, effective history and a physical exam, explain and educate the patient on diagnosis and treatment options, and explain the risks and benefits of each treatment option?

4. Do you feel forced by the low reimbursement rate to do less for the patient than you feel is right?

5. Do you have to hire additional staff to manage the managed health care plans, just to get the insurance companies to pay what they promised in the first place? Is this amount of reimbursement usually or always less than you need to run an efficient and even modestly profitable practice?

6. Have you figured out how much it costs you to "open your doors" with full staffing, per hour (including the staff that has to interact with insurance companies to obtain payment)?

7. If you have, then look at the reimbursement rate of each PPO/HMO you are signed up for, and figure out how fast you have to "move patients" through the doors to break even, including (or not including) a salary for yourself.

8. Do you feel that the stress of running your practice, racing from room to room and trying to keep your patients' histories straight, is harmful to your health, happiness and well-being?

If your calculations resulted in negative numbers, or you realized that the push to survive financially is the driving force for your treatment "style," you may want to consider resigning from the PPO/HMO networks and providing your patients with a fully filled-out invoice that has everything they need to obtain reimbursement directly. Give them claim forms too. You can download claim forms from just about every insurance company, copy them, and hand them to your patient along with the receipt. If you feel uncertain about shifting this responsibility to your patients, you can have a staff member assist them in filling out the form, and provide an envelope so they can mail it in right from your office. By the way, do ask for payment in full at the time of service. Accept charge cards, checks, or cash. The patient will be reimbursed at the "out of network" rate, but now you are free to provide the kind of care that your conscience and knowledge dictate, rather than what the insurance company will allow you.

Perhaps before you do embark on this course, you could write to your patients and tell them why you think this change is better for you and for them. You could tell them what changes you will make that will ultimately provide them with better health care. You can even offer to limit your service to what their insurance will actually cover, but let them know what services would have to be omitted due to time constraints. Then they can decide whether to choose this option and try to get what they need in other ways.

Your patients should also be encouraged to do the preliminary "homework" themselves – that is, to look up all the risks and benefits of the prescribed medications, or to seek follow-up care with a nurse practitioner rather than a specialist. Perhaps they can elect to get the diagnosis only and then look for alternative health care providers for treatment.

Possibly, at first reading, patients will be angry at this advice. They might like having to pay no more than a $20 co-pay at the office (and maybe getting a notice only later for the amount *not* covered by insurance). They might enjoy seeing a note from the insurance company showing them, black on white, how much money they "saved." Problem is, the money subtracted from the doctor's fee is put in the pocket of the insurance company, because they have restricted *the amount, quality, and type* of health care patients can receive.

Health insurance rates have not dropped over the past 20 years since these managed care companies have come into being, have they? No, health insurance premiums have gone *up*. When you, as a patient, see your next EOB (Explanation of Benefits) form explaining how much was "saved" by reducing the fee of the doctor, hospital, or lab, imagine a huckster at a carnival getting you to pay a dollar to guess which cup has the pea under it, when in fact, it was just slipped into the huckster's hand or sleeve.

This kind of pressure is bankrupting physicians across the country and closing down hospitals and clinics (especially any hospital that offers emergency services), because the rates that insurance companies *will pay* are not sufficient to provide adequate staff and medical treatment and to maintain the equipment in the offices and medical buildings. The longer that physicians and patients willingly surrender their choices to the dictates of managed care and health insurance companies, the worse it will be for both health care providers and patients.

The costs of medical care are rising, especially prescription medications and diagnostic procedures such as laboratory and various kinds of scans and analyses. Yes, health insurance rates have gone up, but hospitals are still closing, doctors are still going out of business, laboratories are shutting down and being bought out by bigger labs. Many communities do not have access to specialists, and a number of hospitals have fired the most qualified and highly educated RN's, relying instead on poorly trained medical assistants[3]. Hospitals cannot afford qualified nurses anymore and the nurses do not want to work under such horrendous conditions anyway.

At the end of the day, both the physician and the patient lose out and the insurance industry wins.

Many of the doctors listed on your health plan as "preferred providers" are often no longer contracting with the insurance company. Some of them are no longer in the business. It can take up to two years for a doctor to get his or her name off a "preferred provider" list once he or she has resigned from a plan. Why? I think the reason is that it "looks good" to have many physician names on display for someone considering a particular insurance company. Many of my patients told me that they called 18 of the 20 specialists listed by the health plan and most of them were no longer affiliated. I have heard this repeatedly, or stories very much like it.

Face it: we are not going to make insurance companies become philanthropists, or get them to "think small" in terms of profits. But we do have to get them out of the decision making process that should be reserved for doctor and patient. Of course we should use our health insurance when it covers medical treatment and medications; but the insurance company should not dictate which medications and therapies are prescribed. If you

---

[3] The difference in training is that an RN has a bachelor's or associate's degree in nursing and has done at least a year of student nursing, vs. a medical assistant who is certified after 3 months of training and a 1 month "internship" in a doctor's office or hospital.

are a patient, look around for alternatives. Using treatments not limited to traditional western medicine may actually end up costing less than your doctor's office visit and pharmacy co-payment.

My advice to fellow physicians is this: don't let insurance companies determine the quality of health care you provide. Work it out so that patients get what they need. I will have some suggestions later on how patients can get the most from their insurance, and how health professionals can maximize service while still keeping an eye on overhead. The bottom line is—you have to get out of those contracts!

The physicians/practitioners who have the hardest time doing this are the ones whose specialties are over-represented, and they feel that being in the PPO/HMO is the best way to get referrals. Primary Care providers may feel this way, too, because the trend over the past 20 years has been to push them into a "gatekeeper" role, where they do the initial evaluation and give "permission" and access, via referrals, to a specialist. Primary Care physicians (PCPs) used to do a lot of the work that many specialists do today, including managing their patients in the hospital, with the assistance of consultations from specialists. Now, the PCPs are largely prohibited from managing their patients in the hospital. This may be less so in rural areas, where specialists are not plentiful, but for the most part, the PCP's role has been diminished.

The point of this advice is pretty simple. The primary contract *should be between the patient and health care provider*. Period. It is up to the two of you to determine what the patient's evaluation is for, the depth and length of the consultation, possible treatment, etc. The health care provider (HCP) owes the patient a written statement of what to expect from a consultation in terms of time, examination, testing (approximate range) and fees, as well as payment terms.

An empowered patient should provide the HCP with some specific information about what he/she wants and expects, how much time he/she will need, and be prepared to present prior lab testing, X-rays, procedure reports, previous consultations, a complete list of medications (including supplements and over-the-counter meds), dietary habits, as well as the complete family medical history.

Think about how much better a consultation would be if providers and patients took this collaborative approach to health care. Add to that a list of specific questions you, the empowered patient, want answered about your condition, or about possible treatments. For example, if you saw a TV ad about a treatment for Attention Deficit Disorder, and the guy in the ad acted just like you, you may have decided to be evaluated for ADHD (Attention Deficit/Hyperactivity Disorder). If you think you suffer from this condition you may want to mention this ad as the reason for the consultation, but also explain what symptoms you have in common with the person in the advertisement.

Perhaps take one of the many adult ADHD questionnaires that are available on the web, fill it out, and bring it with you to the doctor's office. Be prepared to discuss your childhood history (grades, performance, teacher comments), which would be helpful in either diagnosing ADHD or ruling it out. The downloadable forms for personal history provided for readers of this book at **http://www.biomedpublishers.com/rinker-forms** or on the author's website at **http://www.stress-medicine.com** will help, but you may want to re-examine what you have written to see if you omitted some important data that now appears relevant. As an example, perhaps you did not mention that all your report cards in grade school mentioned "daydreaming," "talks too much," and "interrupts other students," or that you have been dismissed from more than one job because of being "disorganized" and not completing assignments on time. On their own, these observations might seem too insignificant to write down in your history, but they are characteristic (and defining) issues for someone with ADHD.

The ad you saw proposed a specific medication as treatment for ADHD, but don't be swayed into believing that this particular medication is the only treatment for this condition. That is where you need to take the initiative and explore what alternatives are out there *before* you go see a specialist, so that you are well informed and ready to ask pertinent questions. There are many treatments for ADHD, from changes in diet to prescription medicines. There are other conditions, too, which have the same symptoms as ADHD but are treated entirely differently.

My example applies to a myriad of health care issues. Whatever the particular medical concern, empowered patients will be prepared to assume responsibility for their health care, and the physicians willing to collaborate with them will form a partnership that can revolutionize medicine in this country.

Chapter 11

Patient, Heal Thyself!

My dearest wish is that you will not have to become severely or chronically ill before you learn how important it is to take responsibility for your own health care and view the physician as a consultant—no more and no less. If you yourself know nothing about your health, and do nothing to protect it, do not expect outsiders to care. It would be like taking your new car to the Demolition Derby, then bringing it back to the dealership and demanding repairs without regard to how it came to be in such shape.

I don't mean to admonish you, the reader, because as a rule, our health care system is not set up for preventive care. You are not reimbursed for doctor's visits when you are well or are seeking treatment to stay healthy. In fact, you are not supposed to visit a health care practitioner for *health* care, *but for sick* care*!* Health care providers, too, have been conditioned to accept their role as the dispensers of prescription medications, according to the aforementioned "standard of care of the community," and have a justifiable paranoia of being sued if they stray from that well-beaten path. They are also, as I mentioned before, under an extraordinary pressure from insurance companies to work more quickly and for less money.

If you have lived a "fast food" lifestyle, with very little exercise, in an environment full of air pollution, pesticides, and nutrient-depleted foods, you are an average American. Did you know that, according to a report by the Centers for Disease Control and Prevention, obesity rates have increased more than 60 percent in this country, reaching truly epidemic proportions? Add to that a sedentary lifestyle and possibly smoking, and your risks for heart attacks, diabetes, stroke, and a slew of other diseases increase dramatically. If your doctor tells you that you are overweight and that your cholesterol and blood pressure are high, and if your joints ache, you will probably be offered several prescription medicines and advised to watch your diet. Do you think that you will feel better? Have a new lease on life? Do you believe there is more you could be getting? The answer is yes, there *is* far more you could and should be getting.[4] And the way to obtain what you need is to entrust your health to the only person who really cares about your wellbeing: YOU.

This book provides you with tools to become a powerful patient: using the internet to find information about your illness, keeping your own charts, determining what type of health care professionals you need and how to find them, evaluating drugs and nutrient benefits, and more. In addition, this book will arm you with information about new laws that will aid you in achieving your goal. You now have the right to immediate and complete access to your records, charts, and treatment options (your doctor is supposed to inform you of what is recommended for your condition, and what isn't—and why).

---

[4] Viewing the films "Fast Food Nation" and "Supersize Me" would go a long way toward enlightening you on the dangers of the American diet.

There is no better time than now to become an advocate for your own health.

Need more reasons than the ones already mentioned? There are as many belief systems for what it takes to be a healthy person as there are religions in the world; and many health care practitioners adhere to their teachings as they would to a religion. Some consider you a "heathen" (in a manner of speaking, of course), if you dare to seek the advice of another type of health care provider whose practice lies outside the traditional standards of care. It can be challenging to keep a rational, balanced view when educated people, whom you want to trust, get defensive, passionate, and angry with such issues. This is where the challenge lies for you, the powerful patient, to determine what is hype, what is reasonable, and what is simply ignorance or arrogance. You could be very intimidated by someone who passionately feels that natural remedies provided by naturopathic, Oriental, orthomolecular, or other CAM practitioners are dangerous at worst, and ineffective at their best. ("Orthomolecular," by the way, is a form of alternative medicine that aims to prevent and cure disease by using specific doses of vitamins, amino acids, fatty acids, trace minerals, electrolytes, and other natural substances.)

On the other hand, some naturopathic practitioners believe that all prescription medications are toxic and should never be used. You might find orthomolecular practitioners who only use substances naturally found in the body and never recommend herbal medicine unless they are a source of an essential vitamin or mineral. I am not going to tell you which one is "right" for you, because that is not my judgment call. That is a decision to be made by every individual after taking the time to research each of these fields in detail.

Ultimately, that is the point of this book: You must learn some things yourself, because for each condition and each individual there are several avenues to recovery (just, as in a previous example, there might be several different routes that take you from your house to town). Find out what is best for *your* body, and with what treatment *you* are most comfortable.

Multiple factors influence your body's makeup and internal environment. We now know, for instance, that a large percentage of the population has genetic variations, which make them more or less susceptible to certain diseases like cancer, heart disease, diabetes, osteoporosis, or allergies. That is because this large group of people inherited some of more than 200 genes that might make one of our body's enzymes more or less active. We also know that these variations can be influenced by large doses of specific nutrients or foods. Individual variations like these make each of us biochemically different, and that is why the best answer for one person might not be the best answer for you. What do YOU find believable, valid, and sensible?

You have to learn where to look for <u>objective</u> evidence to make health care decisions for yourself, and to distinguish hype from fact. You have to take into consideration each party's bias when you make your decisions, because only you have your best interests at heart (certainly, as we've seen, not your doctor, drug manufacturer, or insurance plan). You will have to weigh the pros and cons of each treatment: how long will it take to be effective and beneficial, can you afford it, how toxic is it in terms of potential side effects, how urgent is it that your symptoms are reduced immediately. (For example, if your symptoms are not life threatening, you may want to consider natural medicine, which takes longer to kick in, but is less toxic, has no effect on your health insurance record, and often treats the actual problem rather than just masking the symptom.) Many doctors aren't aware of this, but they are required to tell the patient, when they propose a treatment, whether there is any controversy about the treatment, and whether there are doctors who treat the same condition in a different way. Your health care provider may not know this, but now *you* do. Don't hesitate to assert your right to question.

A good example to illustrate this point is the divergence of opinions concerning the treatment of Lyme disease, caused by spirochete bacteria that are transmitted primarily by tick bites but can probably be transmitted through other ways as well, such as sexual intercourse and mosquito bites. Lyme disease has been spreading across the country for the past 10-20 years and is causing many of the symptoms that are labeled as "Chronic Fatigue Syndrome" and "fibromyalgia." There is a growing suspicion that many cases of Parkinson's disease, Multiple Sclerosis and ALS (Lou Gehrig's disease) may also be due to infections by these bacteria. There is a tremendously heated debate going on among specialists in the treatment of infectious diseases about how common Lyme really is and how aggressively it needs to be treated.

I read an excellent medical legal article that advised doctors in both camps of "belief" about the treatment of Lyme disease. One camp (represented by the Infectious Disease Society of America, IDSA) believes that Lyme disease is easily treated with two to four weeks of doxycycline (an antibiotic) and that prolonged symptoms are merely autoimmune reactions, which should be treated only with anti-inflammatory drugs. The other specialized group (ILADS, International Lyme and Associated Diseases Society) sees this disease as a chronic, severe infection, in which the bacteria has cycles of remission and activity and develops hearty resistance to antibiotics. ILADS recommends giving several cycles of antibiotics over the course of one to two years, depending on the severity of the symptoms. The group also warns that co-infections with other blood-borne parasites are common and must be tested for and treated, because they can make the Lyme disease worse and more persistent.

While this controversy remains unresolved to this day, patients with Lyme disease may end up being treated by one camp or another. It just depends on how they choose a physician. The medical legal article stated *that it is the doctor's legal obligation to inform the patient that there are two treatment strategies and a strong debate going on about this, and which side of the fence the treating doctor is on.* Many physicians, however, are not up-front about the dual treatment options. Each side is passionate about its position, and argues adamantly against the other treatment option. A doctor making a referral to a Lyme disease specialist is legally obligated to tell the patient about this controversy and to which school of thought the specialist subscribes. If this disclosure is not given to you, ask; and before you see the specialist learn as much as you can about both treatment options so you can ask pertinent questions.

Similar issues surround the use of vitamins and antioxidants for heart health. The American Medical Association (AMA) has taken a stand that people should get their vitamins and antioxidants from the foods they eat and not take supplements. Many cardiologists have adopted this stance, especially after one study was published a couple of years ago showing that the addition of "an anti-oxidant" increased triglyceride levels in a cholesterol study.

Keep in mind that medical conferences, as well as those double-blind placebo-controlled studies we've discussed at length, are sponsored almost completely by the pharmaceutical industry. If people start taking vitamins and natural supplements and get healthier, and do not need physicians to write prescriptions for them, well...do you see my point? There is no financial gain for drug companies from vitamins. No wonder the AMA is so "concerned" over the use of vitamins and supplements!

Perhaps such glitches in the conventional health care system are the reason why more and more Americans are educating themselves about alternative health care and preventive medicine, and are taking action to prevent and reverse inflammatory processes and treat their own illnesses.

I regularly look for sources that independently evaluate the quality and purity of natural supplements to make sure I am getting what I pay for. There are websites, like www.consumerlab.com and others, that provide valuable information about supplements. I have not yet found any website that lists every supplement produced, but there are several good sources for you to check out.

Make sure the brand of supplement you choose, especially if it does not seem to do what it is supposed to, has full potency compared to other like supplements. I was surprised recently when looking up and comparing green tea supplements that several popular brands contained unacceptable amounts of lead, and that many had very few of the antioxidants that make green tea effective as a cancer preventive agent. I am sorry to say I have yet to find any sites that analyze the real ingredients in pharmaceutical products, and report contaminants, potency and additives. It would be a very useful resource.

Your mission, should you choose to accept it, is to find out if your lifestyle, environment, and heredity and genetic makeup hold any risks to your health before you get sick. If there are, correct those risks. Keep records of your habits and statistics on your health, and write down any worrisome signs or symptoms to watch. (I will be discussing maintaining your own medical record in a subsequent chapter.)

In the coming chapters, I will be guiding you in analyzing medical treatments and discovering their particular risks and benefits. We'll also develop a logical way to make important health decisions by looking at the appropriate use of second opinions and by identifying certain circumstances when it is *not* a good idea to use your health insurance, even if it will pay for some treatments. We will discuss how to evaluate a consultant before you have your first appointment, so that you will know the kind of interaction to expect.

For example, let's say you have done a lot of reading about hormone replacement therapy (regardless of whether you are a man or a woman) and determined that you want "bio-identical" hormones. These are hormones exactly like the ones your body produces. Some pharmaceutical companies produce bio-identical hormones. They come in limited dosage forms, but may turn out to be suitable for you. You might interview the staff at the practitioner's office to see what they know about the prescribing practices of the doctor regarding these hormones. Be skeptical: I have actually heard of doctors prescribing synthetic hormones and saying they are bio-identical, though that is not common. You can see, however, that plenty of pitfalls exist for you, the patient.

I am assuming that you, my readers, will know how to use a computer and have access to one. If you do not, you are missing out on a HUGE amount of information that is now so easy to find. Even kids in pre-school, before they learn to read and write, are figuring out how to work computers to play games. You can use computers without charge at most libraries, and for a small fee at most copy centers, such as Copyland ™ or KinkosFedEx ™. You might want to invest some time in a basic computer course if you are uncomfortable with computers and the internet. Visit **http://www.biomedpublishers.com/rinker-forms** or point your browser to **http://www.stress-medicine.com**, where you'll have access to the collection of links I've gathered to various resources and websites which augment the content of this book. You can buy used computers at very low prices at small computer stores and at computer repair shops. Even new computers can be purchased with all necessary software already installed and Internet access capable for under $600. If you've tried to use a computer before and became befuddled, try again; computers have gotten more "user friendly" every year, and people of all ages are benefiting from them.

Not all health care practitioners will share my enthusiasm, but I am thrilled when patients come to me armed with research and records of previous treatments and a list of questions. These are *powerful patients* (even if ill) who know that I, a health care provider, am a *consultant,* and I take that role very seriously. I want to give them the kind of service they expect and have every right to receive.

My patients are a remarkable group of people who have figured out the workings of the health care system. Over the years, I have tried to teach patients how to be assertive in seeking a second opinion, a consultation, or their medical records. While fighting to receive the kind of health care they needed, many of these "power patients" were suffering from pain or chronic illnesses. Some ended up angry with the medical profession and "use doctors only when they have to." They always come fully prepared to get what they need because they learned the hard way what their rights are and are determined not to waste any more time or money than strictly necessary. They are willing to cooperate with a consultant, but they also demand information, explanations, and a detailed treatment plan. They have been hurt by the medical system, and now they are ready to fight for their right to be in charge of what happens to their bodies and to receive complete, useful information.

They have lost a great deal of trust in medical professionals in general, but consult with us when they must to get the information (or tests and prescriptions) they need. The following story is a case in point.

Zeva (not patient's real identity) is a 26-year-old graduate school student studying design and graphic art, but she has been struggling with poor health for the past five years. During this time, her symptoms, which started out as minor complaints of muscle and joint pain and fatigue had slowly progressed to the point where she could not function without daily pain medication. She had severe headaches, pain and swelling in several joints, deep muscle pain, bone pain, and overwhelming fatigue. She saw many specialists and received several diagnoses, including Chronic Fatigue Syndrome, Rheumatoid Arthritis (though lab tests for this were negative), anxiety disorder, depression (causing this much pain?), as well as Lyme disease.

Zeva's insurance would not pay for the antibiotics to treat Lyme disease, even though she tested positive for the antibodies to the bacteria that causes it, along with three other "co-infectious agents" that are also passed in a tick bite: Ehrlichia, Bartonella, and Babesia (and for which she tested positive for antibody and PCR testing). Zeva has a managed care health plan under which she can see only one large medical group for her health care. The internist there said she did not have Lyme disease, but fibromyalgia instead, and told her he would approve treatment for that, which consisted of antidepressants, pain medications, and anti-inflammatory medications.

With her health declining, Zeva felt she could not fight with the doctors. She was not sure what was the "right" thing to do, so she accepted the treatment for fibromyalgia because at least it was covered by her insurance.

A year went by. Zeva had some pain relief, but she had to increase the dosage of the medications, which were strong narcotics and impaired her concentration. She was wiped out by the chronic fatigue. When she was not in class, she slept, sometimes for 15 hours at a time. She had few close friends, because the energy to maintain friendships was too much for her. What little energy Zeva had, she used to study and get good grades, at the expense of every other aspect of her life.

Needless to say, this was not the kind of life one would expect for a woman in her twenties, but one doctor she visited implied that she must have been exaggerating her symptoms, because how could someone as sick as she claimed to be get A's and B's in graduate school? That HCP never thought to inquire what sacrifices Zeva had to make in every other aspect of her life.

She was eventually referred to a rheumatologist (a joint specialist) and brought her mother with her to the consultation, because by this time she was wary of physicians and their dismissive attitude. Zeva hoped her mom would verify the severity of her symptoms and help her get some results from the doctor. Unfortunately, her mother was as intimidated by the rheumatologist's callous attitude as Zeva was. The physician entered the examination room and reviewed the history he had received from the referring physician. He then told her he did not want to hear anything from her but "yes" or "no" answers to his queries, and proceeded to rapid-fire questions at her. When Zeva faltered, he berated her slowness, telling her, "The questions are not that hard." Then he looked down at her and said, "You are obviously single, and need to lose weight. That is probably a major source of your joint pain."

When Zeva began to cry (and who could blame her), the doctor became irritated with her. He told her she did not have fibromyalgia after touching her lightly on several areas of her arms and asking if "that hurt." He ended the examination by saying she should see a psychiatrist. Without even reviewing the results of her lab tests for Lyme disease and its co-infections, the doctor told her he was sure she did not have Lyme disease. This was a $450 consultation. She paid for the visit without challenging the doctor. However, she was angry and fed up, and would never again let a consultant treat her this way.

After that, Zeva came to her medical appointments prepared, knew exactly what she wanted, and did not allow anyone to speak down to her. She brought research articles with her. She checked out the physician's philosophy and treatment style before the appointment. She demanded that the doctor give her details of all the possible diagnoses that matched her symptoms, and asked how he/she would rule these possibilities in or out. Zeva knew a lot about her symptoms and what they might mean, and she wanted to know why doctors would not pursue certain avenues of inquiry that seemed obvious to her. She recorded consultation sessions. Somehow, consultants became more helpful and more polite.

Mary Vaughn is another great example of an empowered patient learning to assert her rights. This patient of mine had met with a multitude of doctors over a period of roughly twenty years in an attempt to identify the source of her various ailments—hypoglycemia, hormonal imbalances, and serious joint inflammation. Finally, a possible cause of her misery had been identified: a fungus called Candida; a yeast that is normally found in the digestive system, but can overgrow and enter other parts of the body to become a persistent infection. However, Mary had learned slowly (and the hard way) not to rely solely on a diagnosis from one source; she discovered that being a proactive consumer of medicine is imperative to get healthy.

After seeing several different kinds of health care practitioners and reading about her symptoms on the Internet, Mary concluded that one of her problems was excessive inflammation. With further research, she learned that there were many reasons why a person might have excessive inflammation. In her case, an inflamed, frozen shoulder was caused by fast-forming scar tissue, the result of her body's indiscriminating reaction to irritants. Some people have a similar problem due to diabetes, and others because of allergies. In Mary's case, it turned out that she had a chronic systemic yeast infection, and had been suffering from it for years without knowing it. "I came across an article on the Internet that said inflammation starts in the digestive system," she says. "I had some blood work done and the results came back saying that I either had food allergies or an infection, possibly parasites. In fact, it was a bad case of Candida, a yeast infection. I learned that taking a lot of antibiotics or having hormone imbalances can cause a yeast overgrowth. I saw a Naturopathic doctor who started me on a treatment to get the yeast back under control."

One of the things Mary tried to treat her rampant yeast infection was a machine that emits an electromagnetic frequency. When tuned to a specific oscillation the machine kills yeast cells (as well as bacterial, viral, and fungal cells) in the body. This device (usually referred to as a "rife machine") has become quite popular for treating a wide variety of infections where antibiotics have failed. The FDA does not approve it, and people who use it have to do their own research to determine if this treatment would work for them. Mary uses the rife machine currently and sees dramatic results following her treatments, and the improvements last for several days in a row. She also consults with a nutritionist and a specialist in natural hormone treatment.

"I've always questioned authority," Mary says. "With my shoulder, I ended up with lots of different doctors. One would tell me one thing, and then another would tell me something completely different. There was a nugget of truth in what each one had to say, but it wasn't complete, even though sometimes they would think they had the whole answer to my problem. So I started putting things together myself. I read a bunch of books. I guess I have this need to be in control of my own life, otherwise it would get very depressing. When I start having problems, I say, 'I'm not going to settle for this.' I'll gladly go to doctors, but I know I also need to do my own research."

That assertive attitude, Mary says, did not always meet her health care provider's approval. "At one point my naturopath told me, 'I find it hard to believe you're still having problems with the Candida.' She was really irritated that I would question her expertise. It is very disappointing when a health care practitioner meets one with disbelief. After all, why would I spend my money to go there and tell her lies?"

Mary continues to work with several different types of health care practitioners and surfs the Internet regularly. "The Internet has been very helpful. I'm out there still checking out other options. I figure I'm the way of the future; they'd better get used to me because more and more people are becoming aware of the power of the Internet and the vast amount of information out there. You just have to decide for yourself what makes sense and what doesn't, and see if you can find proof for someone's claim or verify it in several places before taking action on it."

There may be some doctors who cringe at the very idea of patients like Zeva and Mary. It might remind them of their oral examination for their specialty board; or perhaps they worry that these patients are gathering information with a plan to sue them if they do not get the desired results.

But it is not like that. Not knowing an answer is not a failure. Patients may detect when a doctor is evasive or uncomfortable and unwilling to admit that they don't have all the answers. In fact, it is a relief to patients when a doctor admits that he or she does not know what is wrong with them or how to make them well, because it frees the patients to find the answer elsewhere or to ask the doctor where she or he would look for an answer. What would you rather hear? Evasive mumblings or something like this: "Mr./Ms. Jones, I have evaluated your problem to the best of my ability and your symptoms don't seem to fit any category of illness I am familiar enough with to make a clear diagnosis. I don't feel comfortable treating you on a "best guess" basis. I'm happy to give you my best guesses, but you might find that another specialist, or another type of a health care provider, will be able to detect your problem better." I know which one I would rather hear. I would respect the doctor more for understanding the limits of his or her specialty.

It will be to your advantage to have a consultation with your HCP that is concise and orderly, and which provides answers to all your questions. Nothing is more frustrating than waiting a month for a consultation, seeing the doctor for only 10 minutes, and never getting to ask the most pressing questions. If you fax your questions to the doctor in advance of an appointment, and have them in front of you during the consult, you can check them off as they are answered, and you will be sure to get what you came for.

Here is the second most frustrating event for a patient: going to a specialist, giving your complete history, then being told that he or she needs to see your previous lab work before prescribing treatment, and scheduling you for an appointment in another month. If you bring a complete copy of your charts from every doctor you have ever consulted, you will have all the information right there with you. It will save time and money, and prevent delay in your treatment. That is why I strongly urge you to organize and keep your own chart, or medical record, and I will explain how and why as we go along. I will also explain to you your rights to privacy and access to your chart and lab tests. It is important for any future treatment you may need that you maintain your own medical record.

It is also your right to record a consultation. It is very easy to forget a technical explanation of something brand new to you. If you have a recording of the consult, you will later be able to absorb the whole thing. You do not need the doctor's permission to record the session, as you are the one paying for it, but do inform him or her that you are recording. I encourage patients to bring a recording device to their wrap-up session when I am going to go over their results, as I spend a lot of time in my explanations, and most people are glad to have the recording by the end of the session.

All of the tips contained in this chapter will help provide you with the practical and psychological advantages you need to take charge of your medical care. Arm yourself with this knowledge and prepare yourself to use it to best advantage. Remember, you have both the right and obligation to become your own advocate and to demand the best health care out there.

Chapter 12

Question The "Evidence"

Many patients are beginning to resist the trend of blindly accepting the dictates of mainstream medicine. It is not uncommon to read widely conflicting news reports about the pros and cons of medicines and therapies. The consumer, however, is becoming curious about health care options and willing to look beyond the headlines in the search for the most effective therapies.

As an example, I would like to cite again the controversial and much talked about "Women's Health Initiative" (WHI) study, which I discussed earlier in the book.

This study concluded that hormone replacement therapy (HRT) was not as helpful or healthy for post-menopausal women as the medical establishment had believed. The implication was that all forms of HRT fall under this broad umbrella. One might even have assumed that with such a huge study (it included approximately 161,000 women ages 50-79), all types of hormones were studied, especially when the research results included broad generalizations about the risks of all forms of hormone replacement.

Reading the newspaper and medical journal articles that reported on the WHI, I, as a physician, was struck by what was missing. Nowhere was it mentioned that only one form of hormone replacement was used in the study. Premarin™ (synthetic estrogen) and Prempro™ (a combined form of Premarin™ and the synthetic progesterone Provera™) were the only three drugs used, both provided by their manufacturer, Wyeth-Ayerst Pharmaceutical Company. These patented, synthetically produced hormones are the most popular on the American market. In many important ways, however, they are quite unlike the hormones naturally secreted by a woman's body. If they were, they could not have been patented, because "bio-identical" hormones can be made from plant products and cannot be patented in the same way as a conventional medication. As we have already mentioned, drug companies profit only from their patented drugs.

So the study was *really* about how Premarin and Prempro worked for post-menopausal women. I wondered how Wyeth-Ayerst, or the spokespersons for the study, managed to get away with not divulging this important fact for several years. There were other problems too. It seemed that many of the women chosen for the study were not the same type as those who usually start hormone replacement. The typical patient begins hormone therapy at the onset of menopause and has a lot of uncomfortable symptoms (hot flashes, night sweats, mood swings, etc). Instead, most of the study subjects were well past menopause and no longer suffered from these symptoms.

Because estradiol (the predominant and most potent estrogen produced by our bodies) *does* protect women from arteriosclerosis and heart disease, the study participants, who were many years post-menopausal and had not taken hormones before, had a much higher level of these problems. Therefore, starting Premarin™ and Provera™ replacement contributed to the formation of unstable plaque, especially in those women who took Provera™ along with the estrogen. There were more heart attacks, rather than fewer. There were more strokes, and more invasive, severe cancers. It is not that I do not understand why Wyeth-Ayerst wanted to spread the blame around equally to all brands and forms of estrogen. My question is, how did they get away with it for so long? And why are they still getting away with it?

Interestingly enough, Europeans, who use different types and brands of HRT than we do in this country, were much more cautious about accepting the findings of this study. They kept a healthy—no pun intended—skepticism. Could it be because their pharmaceutical industry is not as powerful as ours? In Europe, many forms of hormone replacement are prescribed by physicians, including bio-identical transdermal hormones that have been available in Europe through pharmacies for years and don't have to be compounded individually by specialty pharmacies.

But in the U.S., hormone replacement therapy got a very bad rap. Doctors across the country advised women to go off the treatment. They did, and relapsed into miserable menopausal symptoms. No one was talking about the fact that only one type of estrogen (Premarin) and one type of progesterone (Provera), both not natural to the human body, were the only hormones studied. No one mentioned that most of the study group women were 10-15 years post-menopausal when they began the hormone treatment, and that this is not the usual time when most women begin HRT.

It took almost three years before these discussions began to leak into the press, the Internet, and other public forums. Celebrity books, like Suzanne Sommer's *The Sexy Years*, helped to open the discussion on bio-identical hormone replacement as an option that was not commonly known to women. Ms. Somers told her own story of being a breast cancer survivor, and being unable to get anyone to give her hormone replacement as she entered menopause, until she found out about bio-identical hormones. She interviewed three well-known physicians who practiced natural hormone replacement therapy, shared in her book what she learned from them, and how she benefited from their treatment. *The Sexy Years* helped many women (and men) become aware that there were physicians prescribing still beneficial but far less harmful hormone therapies, with fewer side effects and risks.

Gradually, this information is filtering out to the health science community and to the general public as well. After WHI study results were published, women were going off hormones by the thousands. Then, with nothing to effectively relieve menopausal symptoms, they returned to their hormone replacement, sometimes to a lower dose, sometimes changing brands. Many women at this time discovered compounded bio-identical hormone replacement and sought out doctors who knew how to prescribe them. It meant that they would receive a dose of hormones that were in no way different from those that their bodies produced, and that the dosage could be individually adjusted to each person's symptoms, history, and risk factors.

Compounding pharmacies, which allow a physician to order just what each individual needs, rather than "one-size-fits-all" dosages that pharmaceutical companies make, experienced an unprecedented growth in business as women educated themselves and turned to this form of treatment. Is it 100 percent safe, guaranteed not to increase cancer or heart attack risk? No, because there is no "zero risk" in medicine. However, depending on the physician you see, your risks can be substantially reduced by understanding how your body metabolizes estrogens, by monitoring your cardiovascular response to hormone replacement, and by using the lowest dose of the most effective form for each individual's body and response.

Would you be surprised to learn that last year Wyeth-Ayerst submitted a "Citizen's Petition" to the Food and Drug Administration, requesting that compounding pharmacies be restricted from dispensing bio-identical hormones? The drug manufacturer asserted that they were *concerned* for the safety of women who were receiving these hormones without FDA regulation. Wyeth-Ayerst further claimed that these patients falsely believed they were completely safe from any of the risks of hormone replacement therapy.

The petition ignores the fact that compounding pharmacies dispense medications only on the order of a physician, just as any pharmacy would. Can the FDA dictate to physicians exactly what prescriptions they can write? No. Once the FDA approves a medication, it is the physician's discretion to determine the dosage and route of administration that is best for the patient. The hormones in compounded bio-identical creams, pills, and tablets were approved by the FDA many years ago. (The FDA's recent announcement prohibiting compounding pharmacies from dispensing bio-identical Estriol is not because the hormone is not approved; it is because they have not specifically approved a patented prescription drug with Estriol for use in women with menopausal symptoms.)

After release of the Wyeth-Ayerst petition, the FDA was deluged with over 40,000 letters and emails from patients, physicians, and pharmacies nationwide, protesting the petition and any planned restriction of a physician's right to order custom-made, individualized hormone prescriptions for their patients. I wonder why Wyeth-Ayerst did not take Prempro™ and Provera™ off the market after the findings of the WHI, since they are so concerned about the safety of women?

The manipulation of the findings of the Women's Health Initiative is just another example that drives home the point that we must become well enough informed to take charge of the quality of health care we receive. If you want change *now, right away,* you will have to create it yourself, in your own life, in the steps you take whenever you require a health intervention. Big changes often start with little steps taken by ordinary people. If you are frustrated and angry at the quality and cost of health care, your actions as a discriminating consumer and empowered patient will change your life and, possibly, somewhere down the line, the lives of others as well. Many people have begun this process already. I have seen them in my practice, and I know that the "movement" is growing. Join it!

How? To start, all you need is a willingness to become the "healthy skeptic" we described in Chapter 4 and to demand detailed explanations of any medical advice given. Ask your HCPs for alternatives, so that you can make an informed choice. Ask about the pros and cons of each alternative. Don't forget: If the practitioner cannot or will not offer alternative treatment suggestions, seek a second opinion. Do not settle for the dismissive "Here, take this and call me next week," which is basically a twist on the old classic line, "Take two aspirins and call me in the morning." So take notes, go online, and research what you were told. Explore alternatives yourself. No one else will guard your health the way you can.

Chapter 13

Learn What's Good For You

I want this book to give you the resources to learn how to evaluate pharmaceutical drugs, vitamins, and nutritional products, as well as the claims made by their manufacturers. Some doctors enjoy digging deep and researching the claims made by manufacturers to see whether or not there is some validity to them. Other medical professionals either cannot or will not or do not know how to check these claims. Why should *you*? The answer is clear and simple: You must learn about the substances you are putting into your body. Are they beneficial or harmful?

One great resource for people with access to a PDA (handheld pocket computer) is Epocrates™ (www.epocrates.com) software. It is a downloadable, subscription, mobile software program, designed for physicians, but anyone can subscribe. The software has information about the side effects, uses, and dangers of all currently prescribed medications in the United States, as well as many herbal and vitamin preparations. You can also enter into the program the names of all the meds and supplements you are taking and check for interactions. The RX (medications and supplements) software subscription is about $28 per year, but you may also find it useful to get the DX (diagnosis), Lab (blood and urine tests), and SX (symptoms) sections. I use this software every day. The Epocrates website also provides free access to information about drugs and supplements. Parts of the service itself are free, and are also available for the iPhone.

I have come to believe that, while medications play an important role in curing many illnesses, they are not all that important in maintaining health. Vitamins, nutrients, diet, lifestyle, and natural supplements can restore balance in the body and maintain optimal health so that medication for serious illness is not necessary. In many non-urgent cases, it is far better to try the natural approach first—organic substances, vitamins, or herbal supplements. Our bodies process these natural substances much more effectively than the synthetic ones. You should seek the advice of a health care practitioner whom you trust before stopping any medication, but do get several opinions and do research all the medications you are taking. Using the software I mentioned above, or simply researching the matter on the Internet, find out all of the risks, benefits, and side effects.

Another indispensable (traditional medical) book is the *Merck Manual.* It has a description of every condition in every specialty, the means to diagnose it, and the standard medical treatment. New editions are printed every six to eight years. The last edition was updated in 2001. Life Extension Foundation publishes a great alternative health care book, *Life Extension Foundation, Disease Prevention and Treatment* (2003), with updates every three years, which is a similar compendium of every major health condition with alternative treatments listed along with standard ones. Extensive bibliographies are provided in each chapter. Their website (www.lef.org) is a great resource also and has much of the content of both the book and their monthly magazine. Search the online magazine for any topic that is of interest to you and you will find current and archived articles dating back five years.

Yet another good resource is the U.S. National Library of Medicine (part of the National Institutes of Health), which anyone can access at www.pubmed.com. There you can find abstracts (short summaries) of any medical article that has been published in a medical or health journal internationally in the past 10 years. Occasionally the abstract is not available, or it is not available in English, but this website is one of the best compendiums of medical research available.

Using a search engine like www.google.com also brings up medical research articles like those published and catalogued on pubmed.com. But an internet search will also list many other citations, such as online-published material, blogs, and advertising, as well as anecdotal information put on the Internet by individuals. You should be careful placing your trust in information attained this way, but it's also true that even research published in medical journals can't always be trusted as unbiased.

Your internet searches will yield some very interesting information. You might find it surprising to learn how much research is done on herbs and supplements. This particular type of study is often conducted with funds from pharmaceutical companies that are working to identify the active ingredient in a natural substance so that it can be isolated, produced synthetically, and then patented. For example, we do not hear in the mainstream media about the discovery that melatonin, a hormone found in both humans and plants, has the remarkable ability to slow the growth rate of many cancers. However, if you go to the Pubmed site and search under "breast cancer and melatonin" you will see over 200 research articles on that topic. Then try "melatonin and ovarian cancer" and "melatonin and colon cancer." Try several more cancers. The results will surprise you.

Another example is curcumin, which is extracted from turmeric and is the root herb that makes curry yellow. Do the same kind of search on curcumin and all of these cancers. You will find that there are hundreds of research articles on curcumin and its anti-cancer properties. Curcumin has been extensively researched for many years, not only for its cancer inhibiting properties, but also for the antibiotic, antiviral, and antifungal effects. It has also been shown to reduce inflammation and protect the liver from the effects of radiation and other toxic exposure.

Google, Pubmed, and Medline are all useful resources for finding out about the real scientific work that is behind some of these herbal remedies, and also in learning where you can find quality supplements and why one type might be better than another.

If you have concerns about the quality of herbal supplements and vitamins, www.consumerlabs.com is a helpful source of information because it offers analysis and comparison of hundreds of supplements and vitamins, comparing many brands for potency, purity, and digestibility.

When I read that a vitamin or supplement is harmful and want to know if this is truth or "hype," I have found the Council for Responsible Nutrition to be a rational and reliable source of information. This organization, made up of scientists, researchers, physicians, and nutritional experts, analyzes various published articles and offers its view on the objectivity and validity of the studies. Their website can be found at http://www.crnusa.org.

Familiarize yourself with all of the above resources. Use them and other internet sites to find valuable resources that allow access to the wealth of information available to you, the inquisitive, proactive consumer of health care. You, and only you, are the person ultimately responsible for your well-being. It's up to you to learn what's good for you and what isn't, by researching what you are told, by asking questions, and by looking for options.

Chapter 14

The Understanding Physician

I have heard many physicians bemoan the fact that their patients are so passive, that they walk into their offices with the same complaints, over and over, and are given the same advice, over and over. I have also heard doctors both praise and fear the patient who knows too much. If you *are* serious about becoming healthy, and you are getting the same advice all the time, it is *your* responsibility to tell your doctor why that advice does not help you and to ask for a "plan B" (it is called a Treatment Plan, and there should be one in your chart).

If you do not trust the doctor's advice, then it is up to you to find another practitioner who will provide what you need. You can be as skeptical as you want to be about the problems of the American health care (and insurance) system, but you have only one life. If your insurance plan will not pay for the treatment you need, then find another way to pay for it.

You may think that you must go only to the doctor your plan will pay for, but if you are not getting the treatment you need from that physician, the visit may cost you more than you realize, in terms of both money and health. If you only get a few minutes of the doctor's time, and a dismissive, "There's nothing wrong with you," or a prescription for something that will suppress the symptoms but not reverse the cause, then you have wasted your time and your co-pay — and your health.

Perhaps visiting some alternative health care clinics and finding out what their fees are would be a good idea. It may be that you could afford an evaluation, and you could bring that information back to your primary HCP for a follow-up. Think of it as investing in yourself. Some people I know pay more for a pair of shoes than they are willing to spend on their own health, but I do know that for others it can be a choice between going into debt or going to a doctor. If you cannot afford to see an alternative health care provider at all, educating yourself as much as possible through the previously-mentioned books and websites is the first step. Finding nutritional and /or holistic clinics that treat on a sliding scale would be your second one. Some cities have schools for naturopathic, chiropractic, Ayurvedic, and Oriental medical training and often have low-cost public clinics associated with them where their senior students can get a supervised experience in treatment just before graduation. If there is such clinic near you, you might want to visit it.

It makes no sense to keep going to the same doctor if he or she does not offer you a solution that's effective. You may use some of the search resources mentioned in this book to find the kind of practitioner you need. Perhaps your family doctor would be willing to refer you to a HCP within the parameters of your insurance; then again, maybe not. It might be against the rules of your policy. Don't let that stop you. As you have probably figured out by now, health insurance is not there for your health, but to make as much money off your premium as possible. The only way it can do that is to pay the doctor and hospital as little as it can possibly get away with for as few services as possible. Do you actually think that a business model such as the one governing insurance and managed care is going to be primarily concerned with your health?

Don't assume that just because your doctor says a test is "not indicated," it will not be useful to you. Ask why. The doctor might really mean that the test is not indicated because your insurance will not cover it, and he/she is bound by the contract not to suggest certain tests unless you suffer a life-threatening emergency.

The doctor may also be bound by the insurance contract not to prescribe certain expensive medications, except as a last resort, even if they would work better for your condition than cheaper alternatives. There are many Health Maintenance Organizations (HMO's) with such guidelines. Now, even Preferred Provider Organizations (PPO's) send letters to contracting and non-contracting physicians that strongly urge them to prescribe a less expensive medication, or, in the case of non-contracting physicians, that pressure them to accept a lower rate for their services. It may well be that a generic medication will be just as good, or even better, because its effects are well known, while the new drug of the month that is advertised on TV may have some hidden effects that will only appear after the drug has been on the mass market for a while. If you have a doctor who will honestly give you realistic feedback about medications, you will have an inside line on the information that most people would be very grateful to have.

The empowered patient may make some physicians cringe; not every doctor will embrace this new and equal relationship. Some doctors are very uncomfortable with being questioned. Some may be afraid that you might be collecting evidence for a lawsuit, especially if you ask for a copy of the chart notes and lab tests, or if you record the consultation. Some health care providers have a set pattern for treatment of patients with certain conditions and follow this protocol as it was taught to them; they have not explored in depth the why's and how's of your condition, or alternative treatments for it. They may think your questions mean that you believe they don't know what they are doing, especially if they don't remember the biochemistry of the drug they are using or the physiology of the condition it treats.

It would be nice if physicians could just admit that they forgot, and refer you to a resource where you could learn in as much detail as you want about the physiology of your condition or the drug's mechanism of action. It would be nice if they could admit that, beyond the standard of care guidelines for treatment of this condition, to which most people do respond, they do not know any alternatives. Wouldn't it be nice, too, if your General Practitioner (GP) could just let down his or her guard and admit that he or she is not infallible? How can any single person, even a physician, possibly know everything? How can she or he remember the physiology of every single condition? After all, under that white coat is just a human being.

Many smart, well-rounded GPs out there can and will explain your condition to you. Your GP is there to provide the first line of treatment for symptoms and conditions. When the first line of treatment does not work, and if the GP has more ideas, great; but if not, your doctor should send you to someone who studied your condition in greater depth. Some GPs do study a lot and have a wide range of knowledge or areas of special skill they have developed over the years. However, when they do not have that knowledge, a specialist referral is your right. Your specialist may or may not know about every possible treatment either, but should certainly know more than your GP.

It is in both the doctor's and your best interest that your medical chart is transparent (meaning you know everything that's in it), and that you are equal partners in this consultation. By "equal partners" I mean that the doctor, as your consultant, is there to hear your symptoms and needs, evaluate your condition to the best of his or her ability, then consult WITH you on the findings and discuss WITH you the possible treatment options, and obtain FROM you an informed consent for that treatment. You should have copies of all lab work and the treatment plan, if not the chart notes, to take home with you, for your own personal medical record. Pretty simple, right? Chances are, no. The rest of this book is devoted to showing you how to get this miracle relationship to happen.

If you are like most people, you will not decide to take precautions in choosing your HCP until you have a negative experience. I am proposing a sweeping, precautionary approach to your health care. My advice is that you trust no one but yourself to guard your health. Think of your safety and health as your highest priority and focus on getting well as quickly and safely as possible. Yes, you must find health care providers that you can trust, but even the most dedicated and ethical practitioners will not be as vigilant as you should be in reviewing their work and deciding if their recommendations are right for you. It is *your* job to determine if you would be better off with an alternative health care practitioner, though you can certainly ask for the opinion of the HCP you are currently seeing. Just understand that his/her opinion is colored by personal biases, or, as explained in previous chapters, by the rules and regulations imposed by the insurance companies.

If you do not settle for less than feeling well, and you keep your mind open to the notion that achieving health is likely to take several paths, you are already on the road to being your own best health care advocate. Since I started my specialty practice in preventive medicine, I have become more accustomed to patients entering my consultation room with a clear idea of how they want to use my services, what they are willing to pay for in the way of testing (and sometimes it is less than I recommend; but I am just the consultant, after all), and what kind of treatment they are looking for.

Most of the time this type of assertive, knowledgeable patient and I can reach a reasonable compromise. I end up being able to gather enough information to make a diagnosis and prescribe treatment, and they end up with the information and advice they wanted and the satisfaction of knowing that the money they budgeted for the visit was well spent. It is clearly a win—win situation. When the patient and I cannot reach an agreement, it will be because I feel that I cannot prescribe certain medications or hormones without having more information about the patient's physiology, and the patient does not have enough money for or does not see the necessity of tests that I think are the absolute minimum. Consultations I have with my patients seldom come to this kind of impasse, however. The more a patient is clear about what he or she is seeking from me, the better the consultation is. I am filled with admiration for my empowered patients, and it is their stories I wish to bring to you.

One of my patients, Janet, asked that I not use her name and disguise her identity to protect her confidentiality, but she did offer to share her story. Janet is a high-ranking officer in a large corporation, and supervises almost 200 employees in her department. Janet was 53 when she first started to identify symptoms that made her feel "run-down." She was used to being quick in her thinking, decisive and energetic. What she noticed first was that she felt less inclined to go out to dinner or meet friends for a cocktail after work. She then noticed that shopping for groceries and running the usual errands at lunchtime or after work was just too taxing. She started going to bed earlier in the evenings and avoiding social activities on weekends. She relied on her electronic "PDA" for reminders, because she kept forgetting important things.

Eventually, Janet made an appointment with her internist, who ran some lab tests, did an EKG, and told her that, basically, she was fine. He said that the symptoms she was experiencing were "typical of middle age," that she would just have to accept that she was getting older, and that she would have to "slow down some."

Janet was too smart to be satisfied with this diagnosis. Next, she saw a neurologist, who did a brain scan, and said it was normal, and referred her to a psychiatrist. The psychiatrist suggested she might want to try an antidepressant, but Janet did not think she was depressed. Nevertheless, the doc tried to persuade her to try Wellbutrin, an antidepressant that he said helps with thinking, memory, and energy. She took a sample home with her but felt reluctant to take it.

One of Janet's friends suggested she see an acupuncturist/Oriental medical doctor she knew. Janet decided to give him a try. The OMD was American-born, but had trained in China and had gotten a full Chinese medical degree. He was very thorough in his interview, and asked questions that none of the other doctors had asked, such as whether Janet preferred hot or cold beverages, soft or chewy foods, whether she felt irritated very often, and whether she was the type to bury her anger or to yell. He looked closely at her eyes and her tongue, and felt her pulse for almost five minutes. At the end of the consultation, the OMD told Janet she had a deficient Yang, or Chi, in the kidney, and made other statements, which, to her, did not fit the concept of a typical medical diagnosis. He gave her some tea to drink three times a day, as well as three different herbal capsules. Additionally, he did some acupuncture that gave Janet more energy before she even left her first appointment. The doctor treated Janet with acupuncture once a week for about six weeks and continued with various herbs.

Despite this unconventional approach, Janet felt great by the end of two months, and continued to take the herbs for the rest of the year. The OMD also advised Janet to change her diet, as well as her sleep and relaxation habits. She was willing to make this accommodation, and found that she slept better and awoke more energized. She also became determined not to accept the "judgment" of a doctor who says "There's nothing wrong with you," when she knows that there is, and also to search for remedies that may not be part of a traditional treatment but which work for her. Janet readily admits that she does not really know what a "kidney chi" is, but it seemed to her to be something more acceptable than depression, especially when her first treatment made a positive impact. She believes that Oriental medicine may not be the solution to every problem, but now she feels that it is one option she will consider again.

Janet is a great model for what all of us must learn to do in this madcap marketplace, amid the obstacles posed to conventional medicine to properly assess and diagnose, and where even the most conservative forms of health care are full of hidden hazards: the risk profiles for prescription medications; the infection rates in hospitals; or the number of deaths in the standard medical model of practice that are due to "errors."

Yes, even in our country, an average of 195,000 people died due to preventable, in-hospital medical errors in each of the years 2000, 2001, and 2002. These figures were published in a new study of 37 million patient records that was released by HealthGrades, a company that grades the performance of doctors and other HCPs, hospitals, nursing homes, and health plans.

My goal in reporting such statistics is not to condemn the medical profession per se; after all, I am a physician myself. I know there are many excellent physicians who provide compassionate, high quality health care. I just wish that consumers of health care would not put all their faith blindly into the hands of pharmaceutical and insurance industries that define, not exactly selflessly, what medical treatment they are likely to get. Many people are examined, treated, and feel better without any harm done using this model. The folks who are not as lucky are those with multi-system complaints, vague symptoms, and a slow progression of subtle symptoms over time that are ignored or dismissed by their medical provider. Many of these patients do not ever recover or even receive treatment. You might be told that you are ill because you are fat, or getting old, or that it is "all in your head," or that "nothing is wrong with you." At the end of the day, however, you still don't know what exactly is wrong with you or how you can be treated. The health care provider and the system have failed you.

Remember: you *don't have to* accept such mediocre "care." You don't have to accept feeling unwell.

Second, don't settle for a "one-down" relationship with your HCP. In your mind, think of your doctor by his or her first name. Chances are he or she calls you by your first name, rather than addressing you as "Mr." or "Mrs." Yet, you, the patient are expected to show your reverence and respect by calling the health care provider "Dr."

Imagine your HCP as an ordinary person who, at one time or another, might have had to consult a specialist outside of his or her own field of practice. This imaginary test might lead to a mutually respectful relationship. If you do imagine calling your doctor by his first name, let's say "Ralph," imagine too, that he says to you, "Cora, your problem is that you are just putting on too much weight." Cora might feel humiliated or ashamed with "the Doctor" saying this to her, but she might notice that "Ralph" is more overweight than she is, and be dissatisfied with this response.

Take away that power game from docs and they do seem to act a little less arrogant.

First names are not an essential. What *is* necessary is that doctors respond to your needs for information and data. Remember our Declaration of Independence for Health Care? "We reject the myth that the doctor has all the answers. We no longer accept "orders" from physicians. We expect to be treated as equals and to have any proposed diagnoses or treatments explained fully, to our satisfaction and complete understanding. We expect courteous treatment and cooperation." If you follow my advice, your relationship with your HCP will be put to the test. He or she may fail, and you will need to be prepared for that possibility and expand your search for an understanding physician. Or, you may be surprised that your doctor embraces this new relationship. It would give me great joy to hear from people that their doc was cooperative and enthusiastic in their efforts to take charge of their medical records and participate more fully in the care of their own health.

Chapter 15

Creating Your Own Chart

This might sound like I am asking you to be a bit compulsive, and, yes, I am. The pay-off for creating a copy of your medical chart *before you have a serious or chronic illness* will be enormous. The amount of hassle you will avoid in the future, as you visit various doctors, specialists, alternative health care practitioners, or if you require emergency care or surgery, will amaze you. If this is the only thing you take from this book, I consider my effort to write it a success.

You have full rights to your record. With the enactment in 1996 of HIPAA (Health Insurance Portability and Accountability Act), the doctor is obliged to give you full access to your medical chart and record whenever you want to see it and to make copies for you of any part of it. Prior to HIPAA, the patient's ability to create his or her own chart would have been limited. It still might be difficult today, even with the law on your side, because physicians may erroneously think the medical record "belongs" to them when, in fact, it belongs to you. It is *your* medical record, *your* health, and *your* body.

What information should you obtain, copy, and maintain?

I recommend that you start with a large three-ring binder and a three-hole punch (a sturdy one) and put in separators that have pockets in them for small papers, such as copies of prescriptions, instructions on medication side effects that you receive from pharmacies, etc. The general categories included in your note-book should be as follows:

1. **Personal Data and History:** The first entry will be a form which includes all of your personal information. It contains your name, address, date of birth, insurance information, and your complete medical history. This and other forms we will be talking about are available as free downloads from http://www.biomedpublishers.com/rinker-forms or on the author's website at http://www.stress-medicine.com. The form can be completed on your computer, and the accompanying questionnaire will guide you as you fill it in. This will save both you and your doctor a LOT of time in your consultations, because, by writing down your medical history, you have done most of the work of any initial consultation. Just remember to keep your medical history updated and current.

   You may also want to include information about family medical history, especially if there are any hereditary, genetic, or other noteworthy conditions. It may help the doctor with a diagnosis and treatment.

2. **Current Medications and Supplements:** You also can download, from the same websites mentioned above, a form listing every single medication, including over-the-counter medicines, vitamins, and supplements you are now taking. It is important to include the dosage and frequency. Some medical problems are caused by interactions between and among medications; some herbs and supplements are strong enough

to cause these problems too. There is also the possibility of an allergy to one of the medications or supplements. Knowing everything you are taking helps a lot. Modify this list as needed.

3. **Past Medications and Supplements:** This list is important as well, especially if you stopped one of these medications because of an adverse reaction, an allergy, or a toxic effect. Years from now, you might not remember the name of the medication, or even why you stopped it. If the doctor who gave it to you does not have it in the record, and a new doctor thinks it is the "best" thing to try for a current condition, you will be able to pull out your "Past Meds" list and show when you stopped it and why. Your HCP might also recognize in the "bad reaction" list a compound that cross-reacts with something he/she had in mind to recommend and would be more cautious about it now.

4. **Laboratory and Procedure Reports:** Always ask for a copy of any lab report or diagnostic procedure (like X-rays, scans, MRIs, ultrasounds, EKGs, stress tests—to name but a few) you have done by anyone, even if they say the test is completely normal! Most doctors actually get two copies of every test anyway and either throw the second one away or keep it in the chart. Don't take no for an answer. If the doctors tell you that you do not need the report because the result is normal, tell them that you are making your own medical record to have in cases of emergency or for consultations with specialists, and you want to have a personal record of every procedure report and every lab test. Remember: no health care provider can refuse to give you what is legally and rightfully yours.

   One health care organization in California, Kaiser Permanente, has begun a practice of sending a letter to patients with their blood results (minus the reference ranges) typed within the letter, and a brief note stating whether or not the tests were normal. While this is an improvement over past practices, it is not acceptable. Ask for a copy of the *actual* lab report.

One of my recent patients, who does not have health insurance and pays for all of his health care out of pocket, told me of an experience that made him very vigilant about this issue. He had chronic headaches and a neurologist ordered a MRI of his brain. This test cost the patient over $3000. He received a copy of the report. Some months later, when he was consulting with another doctor, this new HCP wanted to see the MRI and asked for a copy. The original neurology consultant said that he disposed of the originals, because he did not have the storage room to keep copies of films for every patient. He contacted the imaging lab and was told that they had also deleted the files from their computer data.

Yes, the patient had a copy of results of the MRI, but what one doctor might see as "unremarkable" on an X-ray or procedure film, may have notable abnormalities to another physician. I have spotted a fracture that was missed by two other doctors viewing the same X-ray in an emergency room. When I pointed it out, they finally saw it. This patient now asks for copies or originals of all labs and procedures *before* he leaves the office on the day of any appointment.

When you have a procedure done, such as an EKG, an ultrasound, or a mammogram, getting just the report of the reading is acceptable, *if* the original records are being kept by a doctor who is not going to dispose of them. Diagnostic procedures and tests are read by licensed physicians, and their reports will have all notable findings remarked upon, and then an "impression" or analysis of the test, and sometimes some recommendations. You also want copies of the reference range (the set of values used by a health professional to interpret a set of medical test results) that the lab uses to report results. Most other professionals, when looking at those results, will want that.

If a doctor tells you that you do not need a copy of your records, you can inform him or her that, according to the HIPAA law, a HCP is required to give you a copy of any part of your chart, and that you also have a right to determine if what is recorded there is accurate. The HIPAA law also requires doctors to inform you on your first appointment that you have this right, and to get a signature from you that you have been so informed. If you do not get such a letter, ask for it and point to the part of the letter that says that you have a right to review and have copies of any portion of your chart. If a health care provider does not present you with such a letter, he/she is subject to a fine.

5. **Consultations and Recommendations:** These would be copies of the formal consultation letters from other doctors and practitioners. Some of them might be about problems resolved, others may relate to your current symptoms in ways of which you are not aware. Each should be a thorough summary of the practitioner's findings.

6. **Research:** This section can include articles you have collected from newspapers, magazines, informational brochures on specific illnesses that relate to you, package inserts on drugs you are taking or have taken, and Pubmed.com and other Internet searches on topics of interest to your health. You may also put here any other information from which you think your doctor could learn.

   Accumulating this complete history of your records is very important. For example, having a record of your cholesterol levels tested over time will be useful to you. When a doctor says your cholesterol is very high and wonders how long it has been this way, you will know exactly when it started to change. I will describe several other examples that I hope will convince you how having your own copy of your medical records will be of benefit.

Example: Saving Time and Money

When I see patients for the first time, I almost always do a thorough blood analysis. Often my patients tell me that they have recently had lab work done, such as hormone and cholesterol levels. Assuming that the tests are recent enough to be useful, I am able to refer to them for assessment purposes. Some patients have a copy of the results of these tests already; these folks will get their evaluations faster, and save both time and money because they don't have to repeat tests. Others have a great deal of difficulty obtaining these lab reports from their doctors' offices. They have to spend extra money and time because the doctor does not want to surrender the results of previous lab tests, or any other procedures such as X-rays, ultrasound, MRI or CT scans, EKGs, etc. (the refusal to release these records to you is, of course, unlawful).

Example: Early Detection of a Progressive Disease

Here is an example from a patient of mine who had a CT scan because of severe migraines. The test was done in order to detect any possible blood vessel abnormalities or tumors, which were not present, but there were numerous "bright" spot densities noted on two consecutive CT scans over a period of five years. The radiologist also suggested clinical correlation regarding the "bright spots" because he/she wasn't given information that indicated that this would be a significant finding. Bright spots occur in other disorders, like Multiple Sclerosis or Neuroborreliosis (Lyme disease affecting the brain).

However, 3 years later, the patient was diagnosed with disseminated Lyme disease. It turned out that the "bright" spot densities on the CT scan were lesions characteristic of Lyme disease in the brain, or of some scarring from a neurotoxin, a poisonous substance that acts specifically on nerve cells. Lyme borrelia bacteria release such neurotoxins, as well as some other harmful organisms. The radiologist had not been told to look for signs of Lyme disease, and neither was the patient given the report. If she had been, she could have shown it to the Lyme disease specialist she later consulted. This would have alerted the specialist that her condition was not newly acquired but had progressed quite far, and could have changed the course of her treatment.

Example: Inaccuracies May Cost You Your Life Insurance

Another example is drawn from the experiences of one of my patients who had emergency surgery for a ruptured diverticulum (a diverticulum is a small "pocket" in the colon) that caused an infection called Diverticulitis. Diverticulitis happens when these pockets become inflamed or infected.

For six weeks prior to the emergency surgery, I was treating this patient for chronic, alternating diarrhea and constipation, and weakness and loss of appetite. Alternating diarrhea and constipation is often seen in parasite infections, especially when it is of many weeks' duration, as was this case. On the day of his hospitalization, the patient was using an enema bag, with a quart of lukewarm water in an attempt to get a bowel movement when he felt a "pop" in his lower intestine followed by extreme pain. He called an ambulance and was rushed to the emergency room. He was feverish, and in severe pain, with an apparent rupture of his intestine.

The ER surgeon declared that performing the enema caused the ruptured diverticulum. I told the surgeon that the cause for the rupture was more likely an infection, which I was in the process of evaluating, rather than simply an enema, which I thought was impossible. The CT Scan of his abdomen revealed a small rupture in his rectum, but it also showed that his rectal tissue was highly inflamed for twelve inches from the anus up to the point of rupture. The report by the radiologist suggested "clinical correlation" on this finding, but since he was only asked to find a rupture, he reported on this primarily.

I explained that the patient had been ill for six weeks prior to the hospitalization, but the surgeon would not consider anything but her initial diagnosis. The patient was operated on to repair the small hole in the intestine, and left the hospital four days later. Subsequently, I received the results of the culture that was sent in just prior to the rupture, and it showed that he indeed had two intestinal parasites. This supported my belief that the rupture was due to an infection, not an enema.

The patient and I requested his medical records after he was turned down for life insurance six months later, even though at that time he was in excellent health, having recovered from his surgery and the infection. We reviewed the CAT scan of his colon, which showed that his rectum had a thick inflammation all the way to the site where the diverticulum had ruptured. The scan also showed cysts in his kidney and liver and calcified lymph nodes in his intestinal area. All of these findings pointed to a possibly significant infection.

Despite all of this information in the CAT scan report, the radiologist's recommendation that clinical correlation be sought, and my own input regarding the patient's diarrhea and infection, the surgeon still reported in the patient's discharge papers that the cause of his ruptured diverticulum was an enema. The surgeon also implied that the enema was significantly more vigorous than a simple, normal enema, and that should be considered "high risk" behavior. This information was simply fiction, but was repeated several times in the record. The patient was astounded. Of course, I asked him if he had said anything to lead the medical staff to believe such a thing, and he adamantly denied it. It was clear to me that the infection was the cause of the rupture, and this patient, who was sick and in pain, was certainly not the sort to resort to performing a forceful enema of the nature implied in the record, nor would he have been able to tolerate such a thing, since he had been suffering lower abdominal pain for several weeks.

Requests by him, his lawyer, and me to correct his record were met with refusal by the hospital staff, because the doctors involved stuck together and insisted that the patient himself provided information about his behavior. His final recourse under HIPAA regulations was to put his own statement in the chart, and to forward to his insurance company my medical records, which documented a history of signs and symptoms of an infection prior to the hospitalization, as well as the culture results proving the parasite infection, and the subsequent cure.

Eventually, he did get a policy, but at a much higher cost for a couple of years, before he finally regained his A-1 rating. The patient would not have gone through so much grief, nor lost so much money, if he had asked for his record immediately on discharge from the hospital, and corrected the problem before there was a financial threat, which made the doctors feel more defensive about their position.

So beware! Not knowing what is in your chart can cost you and your family a lot of money and aggravation.

Example: Detecting Unsuspected Abnormalities

I cannot tell you how many times I have requested copies of a lab result or procedural study which had been reported to the patient as "just fine," because it did not confirm the specific condition the doctor suspected, only to find that the study did in fact show abnormalities that the patient should have been informed about, even if the doctor did not know how to interpret them or had chosen to ignore them.

I had a patient with hypothyroidism, who was told for years that she had "borderline" low thyroid function, and the doctor thought it best to "just watch it" and repeat the test. The TSH (thyroid stimulating hormone) test was repeated four times in a four-year period, and each year the level was higher and higher, and the patient felt worse and worse, yet there was no comment from the doctor that she should receive supplemental thyroid hormone, and a complete thyroid panel was not done.

When this patient saw me she felt like she was dragging herself around, slept 14 hours a day but never felt rested, had lost a lot of her hair, and had all the signs and symptoms of hypothyroidism. Her complete panel revealed Hashimoto's Thyroiditis, a condition in which a person makes antibodies to components of the thyroid, and can have "borderline" and sometimes-normal test results and extremely low thyroid function. She felt better within a month of starting treatment, and greatly resented not being more assertive about her thyroid condition much earlier.

When you do not understand the content of a report, there is no reason why you cannot contact, say, the radiologists who dictated the CT scan, and ask what they meant by any comment that was not clear to you. Sometimes radiologists will see something abnormal that is not correlated to your HCP's specific request when the test was ordered, such as the liver and kidney cysts in the example mentioned above, and will write something like "clinical correlation advised" on the report. This might be an important finding unrelated to the patient's presenting condition. It might also be a "normal" abnormal (something out of range but not really significant), but you may want to look into it later, when you are not in an emergency situation. You might want to compare it to an earlier or later study, if you have one, to see if a cyst has grown, because a growing cyst is significant, but a stable one is not.

Regardless of the particular symptoms, condition, or diagnostic tests, or pieces of the puzzle, if YOU have your records, then you will know if there is a change. It will be a tremendous help to your consultant if he or she is able to look for and track changes. Let's say, for instance, you had a second study of your liver done, say an ultrasound, and in that study they noted and measured the same cysts and found they were bigger. If you brought both studies to your specialists, showing how the cyst changed over time, your doctor would be better able to assess the significance of the problem.

That is the kind of control and influence you need to cultivate in order to become an empowered patient. It will make both your job and your doctor's easier. *You* are the most essential element in this equation.

Chapter 16

Keep Track of Your Visits

This section will help you start the process of writing notes about your medical consults and visits to your doctor. Every doctor is taught in medical school the method of note taking described below, and some of them still use it if they are meticulous in their record keeping. Many HCPs are not meticulous, however, and that is why you might have to push yours to come up with a specific treatment plan that you will understand.

I suggest that you use the "SOAP" format when keeping minutes of your medical consultations and request that your doctors use it too, and that they give you a copy of their own notes (called "progress notes") for your chart. The physician will be either totally annoyed or really impressed by how thorough and dedicated you are. If it were me, I would love you for it!

Now let's talks about SOAP. No, not the kind you use to wash yourself. This particular SOAP is an acronym for "**S**ubjective, **O**bjective, **A**ssessment, **P**lan." The four parts are as follows:

Subjective: A description of your symptoms in your own words.

Objective: Measurable or observable signs of your condition. These are symptoms that you or the doctor could observe (i.e., weight gain or loss, fever, blood pressure measurements over time, laboratory or other test results)

Assessment: Possible diagnosis or explanation of your symptoms. Ask for a "differential diagnosis," that is, two or three possible causes, each with its own probability. A differential diagnosis is of great value to you (if, for example, you want to research the possible causes of your symptoms), and is often excluded by sloppy specialists.

Plan: A description of the treatment plans to be pursued for each diagnosis. Ask for a couple of treatment options, and the pros and cons of each one, so you can choose what you feel comfortable doing. Some medications may scare you, others don't. The plan might include a list of additional tests that are called for in order to confirm a diagnosis before any treatment can begin. In that case, the treatment plan would list those tests and which possible diagnosis each test will help to define.

Obviously, you are not going to have your SOAP notes completely filled out when you get to the doctor's office, or you would not need to see a doctor!

Here is an example of the SOAP format as it might appear on the day of your doctor's visit. The notes are those of a fictional patient seeking a consult with a fictitious neurologist about migraine headaches. The patient was referred by her GP because the GP felt that the migraine headaches, which had recently increased from occasional to almost daily, were severe and accompanied by enough risk factors to justify a more complete and intensive evaluation by someone who regularly sees patients with severe migraines. The patient name and physician name are fictional.

Ideally, you would bring two copies of this form to your doctor's visit: one for you, and one for your physician. You should request that your physician provide you with his or her completed form at the end of the visit. You could re-create the following sample form on your computer and print it out to take with you.

SOAP Format Progress Note

Johansson, Sarah

Age 50, Female
November 11, 2007
Consult with Neurologist Dr. Frieda Beck, referred by Dr. Fred Jones

SUBJECTIVE:

Symptoms frequency and severity: I have been experiencing an increase in migraine headaches over the past three months. They are now constant and daily, some days are milder, and some days are more severe. I get either an aura or a migraine almost every day, nearly always on the right side. I have had migraines since I was about 25, but then they occurred maybe once every three or four months.

Recent changes in medications, food, sleep, and lifestyle: I use transdermal bio-identical hormones and there has been no change in my hormone dosage (recent blood levels attached) for the past three years. I have been avoiding all foods, such as cheeses, wine, and chocolate, that I know can initiate a migraine, and I drink only one cup of caffeinated tea per day. I don't drink sodas, just herbal tea and water during the day. I am not exercising as much as I used to, which helped reduce migraines in the past.

<u>*Previous Medications:*</u> Topamax made my migraines completely disappear for three years. I take 75 mg twice a day, but now that dose doesn't help any more, and augmenting the dose increases the pressure in my eyes. My ophthalmologist said not to go beyond 75 mg twice a day. Now it seems to have no effect.
Current Medications: Imitrex™ 100 mg usually helps, but I try not to take it unless I have to. I take about 15 per month. Sometimes I take a pain pill, like Vicodin™, if the headache gets really bad.

<u>*Previous Severe Occurrence:*</u> I had one migraine about six years ago that caused partial paralysis on the right side. I couldn't speak or write clearly for a day or so, but it completely cleared up. I had an MRI and an MRA at that time (copy of report attached) and they were normal with no blood vessel abnormalities at all. I have never had another episode like that, but I do have auras where I feel "heaviness" in my arm and leg on the right side, the same side as the headache.

Additional Doctor's Notes:

OBJECTIVE:

<u>*Blood Pressure*:</u> for the past 30 days average 98/72; pulse average 76-80. Temperature average: 97.2- 96.9 (low) Weight 160 Height 5'6".

<u>*Hormones:*</u> Lab results: Estradiol level 64, Estrone level 60, Estriol level 40, Progesterone level 9.8, Testosterone total 44, free testosterone 4.5. (Copy of lab report attached). No problems

with hot flashes, night sweats, or bloating. No periods for past nine years.

Previous and Current Medications: I have also tried Neurontin as a prophylactic (preventive) medication, but it did not help. Beta-blockers have not helped either, nor have SSRI's. I have not tried Depakote because I have been told it causes weight gain, and I cannot risk weight gain as I am pre-diabetic and must be very careful.

Allergies: I am allergic to molds, grasses, cats, dairy protein, grapes, lobster, and strawberries.

Time and frequency of symptoms: I tend to get a migraine during the full moon, and, among other times, when a storm front is coming in, when I smell strong perfumes, and when I don't get enough sleep or exercise.

Family Medical history: Father died of a stroke, age 61, mother died of a heart attack age 72. There is also family history of diabetes and heart disease in many relatives.
Others: I have my complete Cholesterol profile available if you want to see it.

Additional Doctor's Notes:

ASSESSMENT

(Here you write notes as your doctor describes his or her assessment. Also ask for a copy of the doctor's notes.)

Diagnosis 1 with probability:

Diagnosis 2 with probability:

Diagnosis 3 with probability:

Diagnoses ruled out and why:

PLAN

Diagnostic tests or procedures?

Referrals?

Treatments:

Risks/Benefits of each proposed treatment:

As you can see, Sarah J. has left space in the SOAP form for Dr. Beck to ask for additional information. Sarah might not have thought of everything the doctor will consider relevant about her experience. In fact, Sarah did not tell the doctor whether she had family members with migraines. Gee whiz, she does! Her brother has them too, as well as high blood pressure, and his doctor does prescribe migraine medicine to her brother for that reason. The doctor is likely to ask questions that will bring this information out, and then it can be added. Sarah does not have to know everything that is important to the diagnosis in order to be helpful. That is why there is extra space—some of the additional information asked for will be Sarah's "subjective" experience and some will be her objective signs and symptoms.

You might also notice that Sarah created a space called "rule out." What this means is that Dr. Beck is being asked to consider possibilities other than the classic typical migraine. Doctors are thinking about possibilities all the time. Sometimes, if they are rushed, they might not consider them until after you have left the consultation. They might or might not mention them in a consultation letter to your referring doctor. You are helping yourself by reminding the doctor to think specifically about alternative diagnoses and to be complete in his or her evaluation while you are there.

In this case, a medicine that worked perfectly for three years, suddenly stopped, and Sarah still has daily migraines. Dr. Beck could assume that the Topamax dose is too low or that Sarah should just try another medicine. However, one of the things that every neurologist should have in the back of his/her mind is that when a headache suddenly changes character (from being under control to worsening) and is constant (instead of once in awhile; daily migraines are not common), it could be an aneurysm or a tumor, or it could be triggered by an allergy, an infection in the sinuses, or the middle ear. When the doctor asks about Sarah's family history and finds out her father died from a stroke, she certainly should put "neurovascular malformation" on the "rule out" list, even though Sarah's symptoms sound like a migraine. Dr. Beck would also want to know what else has changed in Sarah's diet and environment, or if there are symptoms like sinus pain and congestion that Sarah has not mentioned that may be related and pertinent.

It would be so easy for this neurologist to be lazy (especially if she is busy), simply diagnose this condition as a worsening migraine, and change Sarah's medication. I am not saying that it would be a wrong diagnosis, just the easiest one to make, and the one that would take the least amount of time. The doctor could have said, "Try this new medicine for migraine prevention, and I will see you again in a month."

Sarah, however, went to a specialist because she wanted a careful evaluation. She should not have to insist on a procedure, but in the very least she should ask Dr. Beck to explain why she does NOT think Sarah's symptoms are an indication of a more serious condition, and at what point more testing would be indicated. Sarah should also ask Dr. Beck what symptoms would make her think of something more serious than a migraine. That is what a "Differential Diagnosis" is—thinking beyond the obvious, beyond the first diagnosis. It is for this carefully thought out assessment that you pay a specialist the big bucks.

Dr. Beck gives Sarah a prescription for a "first try" medication. If she also has a differential diagnosis, she will have a list of items to learn about and explore on the Internet, to see if they match her symptoms. This research is especially useful if the first treatment does not work or if it worsens the symptoms. Sarah might discover information about symptoms that she never thought to associate with her headaches, but which could sway the diagnosis in another direction.

The bottom line is this: Learn from Sarah. Be organized in your approach to all medical consultations and expect your practitioner (in this example, a specialist) to be thorough. Ask for a differential diagnosis and the likelihood of each of the possible diagnoses. If there is a moderately high probability of more than one diagnosis, you might ask how one would "rule out" (or not) a particular diagnosis.

Too many times, I have heard stories of people waiting for two months for an appointment with a specialist, hoping for a more thorough look at some troubling symptoms than their family practitioner was able to give them. When the appointment time came, they were allotted less than 20 minutes, were handed a prescription, and their condition was discussed in little or no detail. Oftentimes, their treatment was not changed at all. Almost never did they see the consultant's report. This is a common occurrence.

Here are two things you should do when you see a specialist:

First, ask <u>before</u> the consult begins to be given a copy of all notes and reports, which should also be sent to the referring physician (your GP). Make sure the staff in the front office makes a note of that. I have noticed with pleasure that there is an increase in this practice without patients having to ask for it, but it is by no means common practice.

Second, *when you make the appointment,* request a specific amount of time for your consultation, saying that you would like time to ask questions. Do this when you make the appointment, or you might not get it. Inquire how long the doctor usually spends in a consultation. If it is satisfactory, then ask if this includes enough time for you to ask questions; if not, ask for extra minutes. If they tell you there will be an additional charge for that, ask them what it is. If you have insurance, inform them that they can use the V code V65.4 to bill for that extra time and that you will pay for it yourself if the insurance will not cover it. That code covers that part of a consultation that is used for explaining findings, lab work, or a diagnosis to a patient. It should be reimbursable, but most doctors do not take the time to explain, and so they are not aware that there is a code just for that purpose.

Be aware that the SOAP format might not fit at all with the doctor's charting style. She or he may dictate their notes. They may type directly into an electronic charting system. You could then ask them to use the information from your SOAP format during the session, give you a copy of their notes at the end, and send you a copy of the dictated report when that is completed. If the doctor will not use your form, then you use it to copy down the answers to all the questions you ask or are asked. Keep asking what the doctor is writing so that you can make your medical record correctly. Continue following the format of the SOAP document until it is complete and you have all your questions answered.

Most doctors believe that they are performing the consultation for the doctor that referred you, not for you. They may tell you that your doctor requested the consult and that your doctor will get a copy of the report. There is something inherently wrong with this approach; after all, it is *your* health. If the specialist does not understand your rights and feels threatened by your request for full explanations and copies of reports, you can do one of two things. You can state plainly that the consultation is with *you,* that *you* and your insurance company are paying for it, and that, according to HIPAA you have a right to receive a copy of the report. Your other option, if you think the former one will make this consultant too defensive to even treat you, is to nod and accept the progress note that he/she fills out (hopefully) or have them verify the notes you took as accurate, and then ask your GP for a copy of the report when he gets it. That is when it becomes important to have a great working relationship with your primary doctor.

If you are prepared in advance to be organized and thorough in your approach to a medical consultation, your HCP is more likely to follow suit and supply you with adequate information and time. Treat each doctor's visit as a consumer who expects the best product available. Remember that you and your insurance company are paying for a service and that you have every right to get what you pay for.

Chapter 17

Maintain the Right to Review and Correct Your Chart

The Health Insurance Portability and Accountability Act (HIPAA), described in Chapter 15, allows you full access to your medical records. It also gives you the right to review your chart and request that inaccurate or false or irrelevant statements be changed. If the treating doctors refuse to do so, you are allowed to include a 250-word statement of your own to clarify the issue, which will become a part of your medical record.

It is useful to request copies of procedures, lab tests, and reports not only to facilitate future consults and treatments from all HCPs, but also to search out inaccuracies that you will want to pursue and correct. The purpose is for you to be in control of your medical record and the course of your health care as much as you possibly can.

The HIPAA Privacy Rule also provides protection for the patient's confidentiality. There is now a standard form, which most doctors' offices have you sign, which tells you what might be done with the information from your chart. It should be clear when, how, and to whom a HCP will release this information. Most offices download a generic form and many of them are pretty much the same, but I would urge you to read it anyway.

You may not agree with parts of form's content, especially if you want to have some say about what information goes to whom. Most forms give the doctor the freedom to send the contents of your chart to anyone who presents a copy of your signature on a "release of information" form. You sign such forms all the time without realizing it, for bank loans, life insurance, health insurance, employment; and sometimes they do not have expiration dates. It is unusual, and perhaps even novel, for the patient to come into the office with his or her own forms about the release of medical information, but I think it is time that we make this happen.

I have made it my practice to protect my patients' confidentiality for the past 18 years, ever since a lawyer used some potentially embarrassing information, said in confidence and noted in my chart, to blackmail one of my patients into dropping a civil suit. This information had nothing to do with the patient's case as a plaintiff in a medical injury case involving a retail store. Yet, he was forced to drop his suit (for medical expenses for his injuries) in order to protect himself from the threat of public humiliation. At that time, my secretary did not know that when a subpoena is served, the chart does not have to be handed over on the spot.

This was a painful lesson for me, but I learned from it. And the lesson was that I must write notes in my chart that would not compromise the privacy of the patient or any other individual. From that time on, I told my patients that I would never release anything from my office that they had not personally reviewed and cleared, even if I were presented a signed consent. I also emphasize to my staff that they should never, ever, release anything to anyone, even if handed a written consent or a subpoena, until the patient has read the chart and approved each page.

Many consent forms for release of medical information are routinely obtained by insurance carriers, employers, and disability companies, and the patient may not even be aware of having once signed the consent, and often does not know about the request for his chart. You may have a great relationship with your doctor but don't remember that you said some very personal things a couple of years ago, things that might embarrass you if made public. You have a right to ask that such information be removed.

Here is an example of how this situation can come back to bite you in unexpected ways: I had a patient who was self-employed and did not have health or life insurance. During a difficult divorce, he was prescribed an anti-anxiety medication because his mental state warranted it at the time. The divorce dragged on for over a year, and he became physically dependent on the medication. He discussed with me how to get off it once this stressful time was over. We devised a schedule for titrating off with a long acting version of the same medication; he was following the schedule and doing well with it. He would be off the medication completely, without withdrawal symptoms, within a month or so.

Six weeks later, I referred him to a dermatologist for an annoying rash. He mentioned his current medications and the plan we had developed to slowly withdraw the anti-anxiety medicine. A year later, he applied for life and health insurance but was turned down. When he inquired why, he was told it was because of something in his medical records, so he requested charts from all his doctors. Since his general health was good, there was nothing objectionable in his chart, other than the dermatologist's notation that he was a "Valium addict."

My patient confronted the dermatologist, who refused to change his record to reflect the true nature of this patient's "addiction," (i.e., that he was titrating off an anti-anxiety medication taken under a doctor's supervision for a specific, and temporary, condition). This was before HIPAA, which addresses the security, accuracy, and privacy of medical records, came into effect. The poor man was stuck with a medical record that can be a liability to getting insurance, or could cause future health care service providers to be prejudiced. His only recourse would be to wait awhile, start over with a new insurance company, and not list the dermatologist's name, since it was only one consult. Fortunately, today, under HIPAA guidelines, a patient can request to change incorrect information in his or her charts. If the doctor refuses, then, by law, the doctor must also include in the chart the patient's statement explaining the issue, and if records are requested again, that statement must go out with it.

Once a copy of the chart is released outside of the doctor's office, that information is out there in the public (perhaps in a lawyer's office, another doctor's office, an insurance company's file), and you do not know who has or will have access to it. Now, with the advent of electronic medical records, the privacy of your medical chart is becoming even more of a concern. If you do not supervise the contents yourself, I can promise you that no one else is going to be the guardian of accuracy or the protector of your privacy. You must know what is in your medical records, and you must make sure the information is accurate.

When one of my patients comes in to review his or her chart prior to my releasing it to some interested party, I give them a pad of thin post-it markers and tell them to read the chart with the idea of protecting their privacy, as well as the privacy of other people who might be mentioned (the boss, a co-worker, the spouse, etc.). If a comment would compromise someone's privacy, and is not relevant to the issue for which the interested party is seeking data, it should be brought to my attention.

Many times, insurance companies or lawyers have inquired why there is a "blanked out" area on a patient's chart. I simply inform them that the information deleted was not relevant to their inquiry and would compromise the privacy of the patient or someone else who has not given consent for release of personal information. I have never had a problem with this.

I also instruct the patient to note any information that is not accurate or would cause them great embarrassment if seen by other people. An example of this might be someone who is applying for life insurance and had a discussion one day about erectile dysfunction. This would hardly be a reason to deny life insurance, but the patient may not want this note to be part of the chart that sits in the insurance company office to be read by a non-medical person.

Perhaps you think that such scenarios are unlikely events. I am sorry to have to tell you they are common. Not only are errors in histories often made (I make them myself and wouldn't even know it if I did not have in my practice a policy of patient review), but also, questionable judgments are often made by HCPs and not ever discussed with the patient. It is not uncommon for the doctor to write in the chart that he thinks the patient is addicted to a drug or alcohol without ever mentioning this annotation to the patient. This may be because the doctor does not feel comfortable bringing up the topic or does not have time to discuss it, but it is unfair to the patient to put this in the chart without disclosing it.

If you are the patient in such a situation, you have a serious issue to deal with. Not only how to address it with your doctor, but also how to resolve it in your chart. If the physician believes this information is accurate but you know it is not, and you think it might be a source of personal or financial damage, there are certain recourses you have within your HIPAA rights.

For instance, you could add a comment of your own to the chart or report the HCP's refusal to change the notes to reflect an accurate history to HIPAA authorities. The prospect that HIPAA may fine the doctor for an inaccurate judgment, and any other infraction HIPAA investigators find, could be an effective deterrent.

A situation like this might require some negotiation between you and the physician. Remember to keep your cool. Ask the doctor what he defines as an "addiction" and what exactly in your medical history, comments, or behavior led him to this conclusion. Perhaps you might read up on the definition of addiction and discover for yourself if you meet the criteria for such a description. If the doctor misunderstood a comment you made, for example, if you were jokingly referring to your college days and mentioned that you had not "partied" like that in 20 years, you might want to stress that now your consumption of alcohol is less than two glasses of wine per week, and has been so for at least 10 years or more. Maybe, given that information, the physician would revise his notes.

I hope doctors realize that a single comment like this can make it impossible for patients to obtain life insurance or health insurance if they are self employed, for at least the next seven years. That can have a devastating financial impact, even on someone who is employed or owns a business, should they have an illness that requires specialty consultations, procedures, or hospitalization. The relationship between doctors and patients has become so strained and mistrustful that this kind of situation, where the careless pen of a doctor changes the life of a person, and the doctor does not have the humility or compassion to question and correct his/her actions, is all too common. Misunderstandings or misinterpretation of information given by patients has been reported in up to 15 percent of patient charts.

If you are seeing a new health consultant for the first time, you want to start off on the right footing during the initial consultation. Give the HCP a form explaining the limits you wish to place on any release of information they receive from any source, no matter how recent your signature is. In this form, you would state that you wish to be notified whenever anyone requests records from your chart and that you retain the right to review any and all information obtained from your medical record before it is released. Ask the doctor to sign it. Also ask who in the office is in charge of copying medical records (there is supposed to be a designated person) and make sure that person sees the form and puts it in the chart so it will not be lost or forgotten. You might suggest that office personnel write on the outside front of your chart, "Call patient before sending out any medical records."

A *Limits on Release of Information* form is available for download from **http://www.biomedpublishers.com/rinker-forms** or **http://www.stress-medicine.com**. The form states unequivocally that you wish to be notified when a copy of your chart is requested. It should also state that you maintain the right to review your chart at any time to make sure the information in it is accurate and that you will request copies of information you feel would be valuable to have in your personal medical record. *That way, you can review your records before you apply for life insurance, for example, and discuss any issues in the chart that concern you before the records are ever requested.* Then the urgency will not be as great and, if there is a disagreement about the content between you and your HCP, you can make a decision to delay your insurance application while the issue is being resolved.

With previous or current health consultants, you will need to make the same requests, but for existing medical records.

Health care providers are required to give you a written statement about what they will and will not do with your chart information. Read it carefully because they are not all the same. Some of these are a *carte blanche* permission to use your private information as the doctor sees fit; that is, to discuss your case with other doctors, family members, and insurance companies. You may want to specify which health care providers this applies to, and which family members, or you may want to cross that line out entirely and put in "see limitations of release form" for every statement that is too broad and is covered in your consent form in a more restricted way.

A sample format for a "Limits on Release of Information, Right of Review" form is available for download as mentioned above. You can print it out to use in your medical record, modify it to suit your needs, or supply it at the requests of your physicians. They may have some conditions they want to place on it, such as a waiver when communicating with your primary doctor, for the sake of convenience, or in a life threatening emergency, etc. It would be best for you to bring in two copies: one for you to have signed and kept in your records, and the other one for the practitioner's records. Following is an example of this form:

Limits on Release of Medical Information

I have read and understand your HIPAA document explaining the conditions under which you would be releasing information from my chart. I have crossed out (if necessary) any points that I do not approve prior to signing the agreement. I am herewith submitting the specific limitations and requirements to insure my privacy and accuracy of medical information released, and stipulate that only the necessary information to achieve the objective of the requesting agency or person be released and no more. This would ensure the protection not only of my own privacy but also the privacy of any other individuals who might be mentioned in your charts, and who would not be able to give consent to the release of information about them, as they would have no knowledge about it.

I wish to be contacted any time a request for information from my chart is made, prior to the release of any information. I will want to review the chart at that time, to make sure that it contains no inaccurate data.

After reviewing the information to be released, if any corrections were needed, I would request that they be made prior to the release of the chart. If you do not agree with me regarding the requested corrections, I would like an explanation of your reasons.

If we cannot agree on any portion of the chart material's validity, I may request either that this section not be sent, or that I be allowed to insert a statement about this information, which will be kept in the chart as a part of my permanent medical record. (For further information on my right to do this, see http://www.hhs.gov/ocr/hipaa.)

I request that a notation be made on the cover of my chart stating that "Patient must be contacted before any information is released from this chart—see Limitations on Consent to Release Form," so that if there is a change in staff, this request is not overlooked.

Thank you for your consideration in this matter. By signing below, I know that you have consented to implement this policy as recommended by the U.S. Department of Health and Human Services Office for Civil Rights.

______________________________ ____________

Physician/Practitioner Signature *Date*

______________________________ ____________

Patient Signature *Date*

One of my empowered patients came to my office recently and presented me with a form she had devised herself. She is on permanent disability and the disability company periodically requests records from all her health care providers. She showed me the form she was sending back to the insurance company, one that she created, rather than their standard consent form that is extraordinarily broad in its demand for information. I present it below, changing some significant details to protect the privacy of this person.

Fortrana Life Insurance Corporation
Savannah T. Roman, SSN: 888-88-8888
DOB: October 22, 1944

I do not believe that the Authorization for Release of Information provided complies with HIPAA privacy rules. As such, I am not willing to sign it.

I am willing to sign an authorization for release as described below:

Authorization for Release of Information to Fortrana Life Insurance Corporation is limited as follows:
I am <u>not willing</u> to release any psychotherapy notes.
I am <u>not willing to</u> release medical information without restriction.
You <u>have permission</u> to request and review treatment summaries from treating physicians. This information may include and is limited to dates of service, diagnosis, treatment, progress, and prognosis. These doctors include: Dr. T. Rinker, Dr. Fred Jones, Dr. Susan Bright, and Dr. Wajna Bourman.
I am <u>not willing</u> to release copies of my federal income taxes. I file a joint return with my spouse and am not willing to provide this depth of information to an insurance company.
You <u>may contact</u> Social Security Administration to confirm any income on my behalf. However, you <u>may not</u> request copies of my federal income tax returns from them. I have provided them with

this information and they can confirm the status of any and all work activity in this regard.
You may also contact Social Security Administration to confirm the status of my disability. They administer the SDI that I receive monthly.
You may not share any information you obtain in my regard with any other agency that is not DIRECTLY RESPONSIBLE for making the decision to continue with the waiver of premiums and/or administering of claims, benefits, re-insurance, and coverage.
This is the extent of sharing of information I am willing to provide. My privacy is important.

I understand that if I refuse to sign the original authorization provided by Fortrana, you may decline to process my claim. If this is the case, I understand that I have a right to receive an explanation of that decision, and how any limitations I presented prevented processing my claim.

This authorization will remain in effect, canceling all prior ones, for one year following the date of my signature.

_________________________ ____________________

Savannah T. Roman *Date*

This letter is a gift to all my readers from one of my very smart patients. If an insurance company sends a release of information form to you, PLEASE READ IT! You will be stunned to see things in it like the permission to contact your employers, neighbors, bank, credit companies (you name it) to obtain information about you. This widely practiced policy is outrageous, and most people sign a release without realizing what they give away. You do not have to create your own form as "Savannah" did, though you could copy hers or mine. You can also cross out with a black marker everything you do not consent to, and write at the bottom. “The crossed out items are those to which I specifically do NOT consent,” then sign your name.

Chapter 18

When Self-Advocacy Is Not Enough

I have written a great deal about being your own health care advocate, but there are times when you just can't do it alone. If you try, you may end up in a crisis without any support at all. The most critical scenario arises if you become so seriously ill that you cannot make your needs and desires known, or if you are unconscious or too weak to advocate for yourself. Designating someone else as your health care advocate, in advance of any illness or injury that renders you unable to make your own decisions, puts the power to make such choices in the hands of someone you know and trust. This person can be your spouse, sibling or other relative, a friend, or even a medical professional whom you trust.

Using a search engine, you can find a number of sites that will walk you through acquiring the information required for a Medical Power of Attorney, also known as a Durable Power of Attorney for Healthcare. This form will provide you with the necessary paperwork to name your advocate and provide him or her with the legal authority to make medical decisions on your behalf. You are usually required to name one person plus an alternate, should your primary advocate become deceased, disabled, or otherwise unavailable. You are also required to have the document signed by you and by a notary public or two witnesses. You can fill out these forms online and, for a fee of approximately $15, you will receive a legally binding, printed form (once the signatures are obtained). Many states have free online forms available on a government website. Since they are no different than the ones you buy, avail yourself of the free form if you can find one.

In addition to the dire circumstance of your becoming incapacitated, there are other times when being your own health care advocate, as desirable as that is, may not be enough. One situation might occur when you feel overwhelmed by the details or complexity of managing your health care, even if you are mentally competent and legally "sane." This circumstance can occur with chronic and/or life threatening and disabling conditions such as cancer, serious heart disease, chronic debilitating infections, or any conditions which affect your ability to process and seek complex information, sort through options and make complex decisions. This type of temporary incapacity can occur with anyone, and having an advocate, especially one legally authorized by you, could be extremely important.

I can remember a time when a relative of mine had to have emergency abdominal surgery. While in the ICU in recovery, the nurse refused to consider the possibility that he was unresponsive to the pain killing effects of morphine. (Five to fifteen percent of people actually have this condition and wouldn't know it until it became necessary to give a morphine type drug for excruciating pain.) There are other powerful pain medicines that could have been used instead, but to do so required a change in the surgeon's order. I refused to leave the ICU until the nurse contacted the on-call surgery resident to notify him that this patient was still in severe pain following the administration of four doses of morphine. At my insistence, she grudgingly made the call while I watched. The medication was changed, and my relative's pain level went from a level 10 (worst imaginable pain) to a level 4 within fifteen minutes of administering an alternative medication. This was after he suffered unnecessarily for 2 hours. But what would it have been like for him if I hadn't been there to insist that the nurse contact the on-call doctor? He depended on me to protect his interests. This is the kind of role your advocate can perform.

There are other, less urgent, but equally important times when you might want to consider including an advocate's assistance. One possible reason for using an advocate is to help you keep on track during a medical consultation, and to make sure the health care provider does too. With your advocate, you might want to outline in advance what you hope to learn from a consultation, as well as what questions you have and want to make sure are answered before the consultation is complete. Being the "subject" of an examination can be intimidating to anyone, especially when you might be worried about the diagnosis or your symptoms. If you also feel unwell, maintaining the proper focus to listen fully to explanations and be ready to ask questions can be very difficult.

Many times, I have left a medical consultation realizing that I didn't get all the information I wanted, and then found it hard to get in touch with the consultant in order to get the answers I sought. You should be able to say after a consultation that you have a clear understanding of what the doctor thinks is the cause of your symptoms or what he or she proposes to do to find answers to your problem. If further testing is required, you should know what the risks of these procedures are, the cost of them, and how likely they are to give the health care provider a clear answer as to diagnosis. You should also have a clear understanding of what treatment options there are, and you should have been offered more than one option. You should be told what the expected benefits will be of a treatment and how likely it is that this treatment will result in the expected benefits. You should also have been given detailed information about the risks and possible side effects of this treatment and what would likely happen if you chose not to have the treatment. Your advocate will ensure that you receive from the HCP the information and explanation you require.

Who can be your personal advocate?

Anyone you trust and authorize to have access to your medical information can be your health care advocate, even if it is only the information they would learn by sitting in on the consult with you. This person can be a friend or family member or a paid professional. It would be wise to make sure your advocate is not intimidated by medical professionals and is willing to interrupt if necessary, when your questions have not been addressed to your satisfaction. (You might be confused or upset at that moment, especially if you've just heard some distressing news, such as a dreaded diagnosis, and not be able to persist in asking important questions.) Your advocate needs to be prepared to step in for you when needed.

Your advocate must also be willing and able to keep his or her head under such circumstances, and know what information you need to have. It might be that the person you trust the most could be as upset as you by hearing a scary diagnosis, and therefore may not be the best advocate. You may want your friend or relative present for emotional support, and an additional person to press for the important answers and a thorough examination. Sometimes a support person is all you need, and you might choose different people to advocate for you in different circumstances, and with different health care providers.

When you select your advocate, he or she should be made aware of what your desires would be under both life-threatening and less serious circumstances. Not providing all of the information you can about your wishes puts your advocate at great disadvantage when the time arises to make decisions or to intervene on your behalf. Your advocate needs the assurance that he/she will be able to carry out your wishes when you are unable to be your own spokesperson. You and your advocate should also agree in advance about how best to meet your needs under less threatening circumstances. It is especially important that you both prepare for medical consults and doctor's appointments.

1. **Agree on a goal:** You and your advocate should talk before the appointment to make sure you are both on the same page about what you want to accomplish during your consultation. An example of this might be that you want to have a definite diagnosis, or know why that is not possible, and what can be done to determine a definite diagnosis. Try to put in writing what you want to know.

2. **Write your questions down, and bring them with you:** Be specific about questions you have. Don't be afraid to ask questions that you worry are "stupid" or "silly." If you have a concern, ask. Your advocate should support any query you have.

3. **If a diagnosis is offered, find out how "certain" it is:** Many health care providers offer opinion as fact, often without thinking about it. It pays to ask for "proof" of a diagnosis and ask whether there is any chance of a "false positive" or an error, or if other practitioners might make a different diagnosis with the same information. The classic example of this is the doctor who orders lab tests, then says, "There is nothing wrong with you," if the lab test ordered falls within the "normal" reference range. You know without a doubt that something isn't right with your health, because you have symptoms that persist, which you didn't have before. HCPs

may sound very certain in their judgment that there is nothing wrong with you, but they are expressing an opinion, not proof.

4. **If treatment is offered, find out the following:**
    a. How effective is this treatment?
    b. What other treatment options are there?
    c. What are the risks of this treatment?
    d. What are possible side effects of this treatment?
    e. What is likely to happen if you don't want this treatment?
    f. What is the cost of this treatment?
    g. How long will the treatment have to continue, and how would you know when it's complete?

    (The same questions should be asked if a surgery or diagnostic procedure is suggested.)

5. **Ask for a copy of the notes from your appointment, preferably to take with you at the end of the session.**

6. **If you know the information offered during the appointment will be very detailed, ask to record the session, so that you will not miss anything:** (Be sure to bring a recording device, if you plan to ask this!) You can record a consultation if you want to, even if the health care provider tells you that he/she will later be dictating a consultation. The typed consultation will be a summary of the appointment and may not include everything that was discussed, though it is nice to have a dictated consultation also.

Using a Professional Advocate

In some cases, you may choose to use a professional advocate. A professional health care advocate is an adviser who specializes in helping patients make sense of our bewildering medical bureaucracy and find the answers they need to make good choices about medical care. You can find Professional Health Advocates using an online search engine. Sometimes a professional advocate can be very helpful during a hospitalization, to make sure you get the care you need. The advocate can be unlicensed or licensed as a nurse, medical assistant, or physician's assistant; even physicians have been known to be available to act as health care advocates and be present during critical times of a hospitalization or during an important consultation. Sometimes they act to coordinate several medical specialists who are conferring on your problem.

Professional advocates can offer many other services, not least of which is assistance with your insurance plan. They can help you file complaints and appeal insurance denials, and advise you through the appeals process. Some advocacy organizations are run by local and state governments and some are private companies that charge a fee for the service, sometimes along with a membership fee. Some identify themselves as non-profit organizations, assisting people who feel they are discriminated against because of race or socio-economic status or who are uninsured or under insured. I have found organizations that assist in helping people obtain disability benefits, through State Disability programs (SDI), Social Security Disability (SSDI), and Supplemental Security Income (SSI).

You have certain legal rights regarding your own physician's duty toward you, and these responsibilities are spelled out in legal terms as to when such obligation begins. The following is from the California Medical Association and the California organization of Citizens for the Right to Know. This brochure is an outline of what rights you have as a member in a Health Maintenance Organization (HMO).

www.dmhc.ca.gov Right To Know:

"Your Partner: (Your Physician)"
By law, you are considered to have a patient/physician relationship once any of the following conditions are met:
1. You have chosen a primary care physician and he/she has begun to receive capitation payments on your behalf.
2. You have spoken to a physician by phone and they have agreed to see you.
3. You enter a physician's examination room.
4. You have received a referral for consultation, and have been given an appointment.

It is your physician's duty to act on your behalf as your advocate for quality care, but in today's managed care environment a physician is allowed (on average) 12 minutes per patient for an examination. That's hardly enough time for bonding, but establishing a good relationship with your physician and communicating your health care wishes openly is a vital part of receiving quality care. Your first and best line of defense during a delay or denial by your HMO of a recommended treatment is direct contact between your physician and your managed care plan on your behalf. Should you need to go further and file a formal appeal to your HMO, documentation from your physician supporting your recommended treatment is very helpful.

It is against the law for a health plan to prohibit a physician from talking freely with you regarding your treatment options. This includes those options that are not covered by your health care plan, and/or those treatments that are considered experimental. Your health plan is not required, however, to pay for any treatment specifically excluded in your Explanation of Benefits.

Above all, it's very important that you understand everything there is to know about your medical condition and ask what alternative treatments are available in addition to what your physician has recommended. Ask your doctor:
1. Why he/she would recommend one treatment over another.
2. What risk factors should be considered.
3. When it would be appropriate to consider another form of treatment.
4. Make sure that your physician will be available to you by phone if you have additional questions after leaving the office.

The brochure not only lists your rights as a patient, it is also serves as a useful guideline for what you should assume regarding the responsibilities of your physician or other health care provider. That does not mean that you are guaranteed these things *will* happen, or that your physician is even aware of his/her responsibility. Many physicians in HMO contracts have a conflict between their legal responsibility to you and the

HMO's pressure to reduce health care costs by not recommending costly drugs or procedures.

A Conversation with a Professional Health care Advocate

I interviewed Kevin Flynn from www.healthcareadvocates.com, and he gave me his view of how best to utilize the services of a professional health care advocate, and what to watch out for. He cautioned potential clients of a health care advocate to be wary of organizations that present themselves as your advocate, when in fact they work for one or more health insurance companies. Why would it be a problem to use such an advocate? As Mr. Flynn says, "How likely is it that someone having a contract with an insurance company is going to fight hard for *your* rights? They comply with the limits that company sets on them. If a health advocate has contracts with insurance companies, are they really going to do what's best for you or for their client?" I wondered how one could tell if an advocacy organization is a branch of a health insurance company, and Mr. Flynn informed me that the only way to know is to ask. Legally they are required to tell you, but they are not required to put this information in their advertising materials. When looking for an advocate, one should ask directly if that advocate or company has any relationships or contracts with any insurance companies.

Another issue Flynn warned about is reliability. He said you should look for a company that has the availability of many different experts and has been in the business for more than a couple of years. It's good, he says, to develop a relationship with an advocate company, so that they know what issues you have dealt with and what your needs are. "Say you hire a nurse as an advocate. What if you need surgery and she is not familiar with hospital procedures, because most of her experience is with outpatient work? Or what if he or she is good at getting reimbursement for medical care from insurance, but doesn't know anything about how to evaluate a good nursing home, or what the going rate for nursing homes is in your area? That's why it's good to have access within the company to people with a wide variety of skills to meet your changing needs."

Health care advocacy companies promote themselves as helping with a wide variety of issues: billing issues with physicians, insurance claims and appeals, second opinions and finding out about alternative procedures available, finding a specific type of specialist, and finding a nursing home or rehabilitation center. Mr. Flynn said that at his company, there are several people who were formerly insurance company employees, and they report that most insurers are more likely to pay attention to an appeal or complaint when they see it presented by a professional advocate rather than written by the patients themselves. Flynn believes that explains at least part of the greater success rate in getting appeals settled by using advocate companies.

The company Mr. Flynn works for is nationwide, independently owned and operated since 1996. He says there are about four to six such large independent companies in the country, as well as many smaller organizations. To get an idea of what it would cost to use an advocate from such a company, I asked for an estimate of cost for a number of different situations which are outlined below.

Cost of membership in healthcareadvocates.com	**$19.95/year**
Cost to find a nursing home (depends on amount of research needed)	**$100-$400**
Cost for handling unpaid insurance claims (depends on complexity and amount of claim)	**$50-$400**

Most services are in this range of $50 to $400. Kevin Flynn differed with me on the issue of bringing a professional advocate with you if you feel you might not get full benefit from a medical consultation. He felt that doing so would alienate the physician. "We don't suggest someone going with you; the doctor will more likely practice defensive medicine rather than practice both the science and art of medicine. He or she will worry about litigation and might be overly cautious about suggesting alternative treatments even if he believes they are better. He might be overly cautious about suggesting an 'off-label' drug for a condition, even if he does recommend it in other circumstances. The doctor might be less likely to venture from the accepted standard of care. It might limit the doctor's honesty." Instead, Mr. Flynn suggested having a list of questions to bring to the appointment, and making sure those questions are answered.

This is a reasonable concern and should be weighed against the benefit of having a second set of ears to hear what is being said during a complex medical visit. Sometimes the best health care providers in the area do happen to have such fears and may not provide the best service they can if they feel threatened. In such a circumstance, if you as the patient feel you really must have someone with you to support you in getting all of the information you want and need, then perhaps this would be a situation where a friend or family member would best serve. This solution is very common and would certainly seem far less threatening to a health care provider.

I have no personal experience with healthcareadvocates.com, nor do I know anyone personally who has used their services; therefore I cannot say that I recommend their service. I do, however, thank Mr. Flynn for his time in providing information about his company and about using professional advocates.

Advocacy Websites

http://www.dmhc.ca.gov/dmhc_consumer/fr/fr_resources.asp#specific
This website gives a list of national and regional government and private organizations offering information and support for a wide variety of conditions, age groups, financial and social situations, and support systems. This listing is for California, though many of the sites listed are national organizations. Doing a search for your state and "health advocacy" should get you a solid list of similar organizations for more specific information in your area.

http://www.pnhp.org/news/2007/august/singlepayer_healthc.php
This is a website for an organization called Physicians for a National Health Program. You can read about the problems with private health insurance and the greater than 40 million Americans who have no health insurance at all. If you are a physician, you can join this organization and help promote the concept that a national health care plan is not socialism but is in fact a desperately needed alternative to our current health care system, one that is generating tremendous profits for drug companies and HMO's and creating the worst health care crisis our nation has ever known.

Chapter 19

"Undeifying" The Physician

Doctors are often seen as deities.

There is a joke that I have seen more than once in medical presentations: "What's the difference between God and doctors? God knows He's not a doctor."

Still, many physicians' belief that they are somehow superior to the rest of us is no laughing matter.

In an online survey conducted to help me prepare for this book, one of my patients posted a questionnaire on his health related website asking what consumers like most about good doctors, what they dislike, and what would they do differently now that they know more about the health care system?

I wish I could tell you that I received a lot of information about what great doctors do, but based on the responses so far, the medical profession is not getting such good grades from the public. Time after time, patients have said, that "Doctors do not listen" or "They do not accept that I know anything about my own body." Many patients report that "doctors are mostly narrow-minded, and hostile if you consider seeking a second opinion," and wish they "had realized earlier that doctors are not always right." "Doctors think they are God and dispense treatment like commandments that must be obeyed." Patients commonly wish that they hadn't been so intimidated by doctors and had trusted their instincts more, and they stated that such mistakes caused them to waste much time and money.

It is crucial that physicians begin to see themselves as their patients see them—as fallible. But more important than that, people need to see physicians as nothing more than imperfect humans like the rest of us, who have memorized a set of rules (which were researched making certain assumptions about the structure and function of the body), and learned how to diagnose and treat certain conditions. More and more people are educating themselves about their health and their rights, and do not want their doctors to look down on them.

The pressures placed on physicians by the insurance industry to limit the cost of service, so that insurance company's profits increase, have pushed many hospitals and doctors into bankruptcy. On the other hand, complying with these demands requires a decrease in the time given to patients, as well as in the overall quality of care.

But even if a doctor does not accept health insurance contracts, that does not necessarily mean that he/she will give the patients quality time, treat them as partners in the consultation process, or be open with medical records. It only means that this particular physician created an environment where the insurance company cannot dictate its terms and rates. You will have to do your homework about this doctor by questioning the staff, through a personal recommendation from someone who has experience with this doctor, or via such websites as www.RateMDs.com that allow patients to rate the quality of a physician's care anonymously.

There are pluses and minuses to anonymous evaluation websites. One patient might harbor subjective resentment and use this website to vent several times using different email accounts. And it is not inconceivable that doctors could pad their positive comments. I hope that more free websites like these, which allow ordinary folks to share their experiences honestly with everyone, would show up, because we do need some way to evaluate good doctors. Doctors who are not just academically good, but good at listening, good at explaining, and are respectful not only of your opinions and needs but also of methods of treatment other than their own. The greater the number of comments on any particular physician, the greater the chance that several real patients have offered their candid view of the care they received.

Many physicians have become either too harried or too comfortable in their positions to recognize that the people they see in their offices are not just "patients" but also customers. The more that empowered patients learn about their rights, the more quality and consideration they will demand from their physicians. This is only fair. The dilemma that many health care providers face, even if they want to provide respectful and open communication with their patients, is time and cost. Most physicians are barely making their bills. The myth of the "rich doctor" is dead. In undeifying the physician, I wish to help the reader see the doctor as simply a human being who should be taken off the pedestal for the sake of everyone concerned, including the doctor's. I also hope that we can proactively create a new type of an equitable relationship between the doctor and the customer. Arrogance, defined as "a strong feeling of proud self-importance that is expressed by treating other people with contempt or disregard," should have no place in a relationship between a doctor and a patient.

You may wonder if the description I presented above is a fair assessment of how patients perceive physicians. In a 2004 power point presentation published online by Andrew Shuman, M.D., for Bioethics Grand Rounds, Dr. Shuman stated that an online search on "physician arrogance" elicited 38,000 hits on a popular Internet search engine. I did my own a search in September of 2007 on "physician arrogance" and elicited 292,000 hits! Does this mean that the problem has grown substantially since 2004, or that more people are complaining about it? Borrowing again from Dr. Shuman's presentation, he cites an article by Allan Berger in the 2002 Bulletin New York Academy of Medicine (Vol. 77, no. 2: pp 145-7). This article defines physician arrogance as *"Lack of proper respect, consideration, and good manners toward patients, nurses, and other ancillary staff; failure to pause, listen, and share a friendly word or two; being abusive or critical of subordinates, sometimes even in the patient's presence; and (for male physicians) addressing women condescendingly..."* This arrogance takes other forms too, and in the 1980 New England Journal of Medicine, F.J. Ingelfinger defined it as, "An arbitrary, authoritarian pronouncement based on half-knowledge and on an unacknowledged ignorance of overall effects."

It is clear by looking at these and many other writings on the topic, that not only are patients aware of this troubling tendency in physicians, but also that some physicians themselves are beginning to see their attitudes as an obstacle to good patient care and communication.

Researchers at Baylor College of Medicine (BCM) in Houston have been studying the evolution of doctor-patient dynamics and ways of improving communication between medical professionals and their patients. Dr. Paul Haidet, assistant professor of medicine at BCM and a staff physician at the Michael E. DeBakey Veterans Affairs Medical Center in Houston, is among those researchers.

I interviewed Dr. Haidet for this book concerning this all-important issue. This is what he told me:

"Increasing numbers of patients are proactive, empowered by the Internet, and want to have partnerships with their doctors, so physicians today must be more flexible and sensitive than ever before. While some studies show that certain patients (especially elderly males) want the doctor to be in control, the majority of patients want a partnership. To obtain that kind of equitable relationship, patients should clearly communicate to the doctor the essence of their concerns and negotiate a relationship they want to have. Doctors can help by asking open-ended questions to allow patients to tell their stories and express concerns. The patient should have very clear expectations and communicate them to the physician. The 'doctor knows best' attitude is no way of getting that relationship."

Haidet concludes, "If the physician is not responsive to that kind of approach, the patient should consider getting a new doctor."

I think most health care providers, especially the arrogant ones, do not see themselves that way. But the perceived arrogance of the physician is the major stumbling block to good communication between the patient and the HCP. If physicians knew how they come across to their patients, and how their "holier-than-thou" attitude is harming the relationship, I would hope that they would change. Health care practitioners would do well to regularly ask their staff to observe how patients react after appointments. Anonymous surveys may be even better as they would probably elicit the most honest responses.

Here are some of the questions that physicians should ask their staffs:

1. Do patients have complaints about the practitioner's manner or communication style?

2. Do they have any complaints about the information or lack of information given?

3. Do they express any dissatisfaction with their treatment recommendations?

4. Do any patients complain that they were not given enough time or attention?

If a patient has the courage to tell the staff these things, it is an extremely valuable piece of information to the HCP. (Of course, doctors might want to ask themselves why these patients don't feel comfortable sharing their concerns directly with them.) If you are a health care provider, it may be easy to think that the "complainer" was needy or excessively demanding, but it is very likely that for every voiced complaint there are several more people who feel exactly the same way but have not verbally expressed their dissatisfaction. They will very likely express their negative opinions to anyone who asks them about your practice, though. And that is certainly not the kind of "recommendation" any doctor wants.

If you, the patient, are "stuck" with a doctor whose bedside manner leaves a lot of room for improvement, then you owe it to yourself (and to other patients too) to let the staff know how you feel about the service. If you are willing to share these concerns with the doctor as well, all the better. You may not get immediate results, but if enough people let the HCP know about their dissatisfaction with the treatment or service, this action may yield positive results.

Patient feedback, even the angry/negative kind, has been very valuable to me. When patients feel that I have taken too long to return a call, or that my explanations of their conditions were too complicated and confusing, I really do appreciate knowing that. I assume that this patient speaks for at least five others who have had that same experience but were silent about it. I always try to find a solution.

Okay, maybe there are doctors who will sneer at you for complaining. In that case, I suggest you take your feedback to www.RateMDs.com. Sooner or later, these HCPs will find out that they do have a lot to lose when they disregard or disrespect their patients. Also, while you are visiting the site, put in some good evaluations for any practitioner with whom you have had a positive experience. If 10,000 people read this book and enter evaluations on every doctor they have seen in the past five years, that website will be jam-packed with useful information for all of us. Such is the power of the Internet!

Another time not to hold back your assessment of quality of care is when you have decided no longer to see a certain physician. Tell him or her why. Compose a letter to the HCP with specifics about how you were treated by the staff, how you felt the medical evaluation was conducted, how you thought your legal rights were responded to, and why you have decided not to continue with treatment.

It's possible that the physician will attempt to get back at you for your honest feedback. One important way to protect yourself is to include in your letter, on a separate page, the form "Revocation of Consent to Release Medical Information." You can download it from http://www.biomedpublishers.com/rinker-forms or http://www.stress-medicine.com so that you can personalize it, but here is the basic text:

Revocation of Consent to Release Medical Information

To: Dr. X
123 Main Street, Suite 123
Sioux City, Iowa

Date: ______________

Dear Dr X,

As of the above date, I hereby revoke all prior signed consents to release medical information to any entity, including insurance companies, other providers, family members, or legal entities. Even if you receive a request that has a copy of my signature, do not release any information from this chart.

This Revocation of Consent to Release Information includes any written or verbal information about me or my records, as well email communications. It will remain in effect indefinitely, unless I personally contact you to request otherwise.

Sincerely,

(Your name)

Why the caution? Dr X might react to your criticism of him/her by complaining about you to other doctors. This is a clear ethical violation and a violation of your privacy rights as well. He or she may write a note in the chart after you have terminated treatment as a defensive maneuver, fearing that you might sue him or her. Unfortunately, these notes could affect your ability to be reimbursed by insurance, or compromise your treatment from other providers. Most doctors would not go that far, but the damage that can be done to you, if such false "history" is recorded and subsequently sent to other places, would cause you tremendous hassle to "undo." Often such errors cannot be remedied at all, so do take all the necessary precautions to avoid this scenario.

If you have decided to terminate your relationship with a doctor, this is the only power you have to "seal" your chart and deny permission for any information to leave the office. Keep in mind that such a letter does not prevent you from requesting a copy of your chart; it only means a doctor cannot release the information or discuss your case with anyone else.

This caution must be balanced with the reassurance that your doctor is a person, just like you. Sometimes actions that you perceive as arrogance may be due to the HCP's being distracted, overworked, or worried about making ends meet in his or her practice. Who knows? Maybe the doctor doesn't feel well. It can happen! When you mention to the doctor or the staff that you are not getting what you need, start with the assumption that your HCP is not doing anything deliberate to insult you. Assume that the physician does not realize how he/she is coming across or truly does not understand your requests. In other words, give your doctor the benefit of the doubt. I would recommend this approach unless the doctor's behavior is so outrageous or insulting that you feel certain that giving the "benefit of the doubt" would only cause you to feel further humiliation and insult.

Chapter 20

Doctors Don't Have All the Answers

Health care providers may react with delight to your systematically assertive yet courteous approach to the consult. (Since my patients have shown me by example what works for them, I am happy when they come prepared this way, and will suggest one patient's good idea to the next. Hence, this book!) They might also react with suspicion and fear, worrying that you are collecting "evidence" and could use it against them. You might think it is not your job to reassure the doctor, but if you realize that your relationship is an equal one, then understanding that the physician is vulnerable to lawsuits that could damage or destroy his or her practice may help you understand what you might see as a bit of paranoia.

The HCP's best defense against a lawsuit is open communication with the patient, a *transparent chart,* and a willingness to receive feedback with humility and responsiveness. If I have doubts about a diagnosis or the advisability of a particular treatment, I tell the patient what I do and do not know about the possible consequences of each course. We weigh the pros and cons together, and then decide which treatment is preferable. Sometimes patients look at me with surprise and exclaim, "How do you expect me to help you decide this? You're the doctor! You're supposed to know what's best!" I reply that I expect *them* to help *me* decide because it is their body and there isn't only one perfect treatment, but several options.

I want to explain to my patients why it would be difficult for me to choose which potential side effect they would rather have. For example, natural therapies are often the best first treatment, but "all natural" treatments may take a while to reduce symptoms, and there can be significant risk of the patient's health worsening in the meantime. These kinds of decision dilemmas are present every day for a physician. Many times, rather than explain all the options and discuss the pros and cons of each choice, the doctor simply selects the treatment he or she is most comfortable and familiar with, and presents just this one option to the patient.

Is that laziness or arrogance? Is it because the HCP thinks you do not want to be bothered with all the explanations of the various possible treatment choices? Does he/she think you won't understand them? Could it be because the doctor doesn't have time to explain, answer questions, and walk you through the decision-making process? Or could it be because the doctor has samples of one medicine and not the others, and thinks you will appreciate getting a free "start" on the medication? Perhaps it's even because some patients are afraid to take responsibility for their health and would rather be told what to do. Any one of these answers could be true and may explain why HCPs take the shortcut from the interview to treatment, without acknowledging that the patient visit is a consultation. A real consultation should have a discussion time allotted where impressions are shared, questions are asked, possible courses of action are discussed, and your preferences are elicited.

Recently I was doing a consultation with a woman about headaches, stress, and severe muscle spasms. We had discussed at length her evaluation, and I had a list of possible treatments outlined for her. Among them were some types of exercise and relaxation techniques, as well as medications or supplements that would reduce muscle spasm. I also discussed with her the possibility that food allergies were contributing to her symptoms. She listened attentively, and we wrote up a treatment plan. At the very end of the consultation she blurted out, "Couldn't you also prescribe some massage therapy for me? If someone would just rub these muscles or put heat on them, that would help me!" I could see by the look on her that she thought this was just wishful thinking, and that I would not or could not do as she asked. I replied, "Of course I can. We can get a Physical Therapy assessment for you and I can recommend massage therapy, ultrasound, and hot packs or cold packs, as the assessing physical therapist recommends. No problem." She did not believe that she would get what she needed merely by asking for it. I am glad that she jokingly (or despairingly) let out her idea of what she felt would be an important addition to her treatment. I agreed with this excellent idea, which sped up her recovery considerably.

Why didn't I suggest this myself? At that moment, it just didn't occur to me. I am the type of doctor who would normally make such a recommendation. Just because a treatment that you were hoping would be offered isn't mentioned, it is not a reason to assume that it's not possible to have it. It is always worth asking for what you think you need or want to feel well.

Doing so would be even more pertinent if you think the HCP's advice is inadequate. For example, a doctor tells you that your joints wouldn't hurt so much if you would lose some weight. And that's that. You might feel humiliated and frustrated because your pain is not being addressed. Rather than patronize you, the doctor should be asking about your diet, your willingness or efforts to lose weight, and whether or not you need assistance with this endeavor. (Not only should the HCP be asking about your diet because of weight issues, but also because there are many foods that increase inflammation, such as dairy products, gluten from grain, and saturated fats found in red meats.) At this point, you might say, "Of course I need help! Do you think I enjoy being 75 pounds overweight?"

There are many possibilities, which the doctor could recommend, such as a nutritional consultation, and/or a medical consult with a Bariatric physician (yes, there are doctors who specialize in weight loss and obesity management). You might need to have your hormones checked as imbalances in cortisol, estrogen, progesterone, testosterone, and thyroid hormones can all result in excess weight. You may also have insulin resistance, which makes it very hard to lose weight and requires a specific type of diet to reverse. Perhaps you have an eating disorder and binge on foods uncontrollably. (A food binge is typically described as eating over 3,000 calories in one sitting, or eating many servings of some food until you are so stuffed you don't feel well). This too is a treatable condition, and is almost impossible to tackle alone. Whatever the reason, a doctor is mistreating you if he or she offers you nothing but advice to "lose weight," when you obviously have a medical problem that is caused or made worse by that extra weight. That is a good time to demand a treatment plan for weight loss, or a work-up for causes.

You have just as much right to feel medically abandoned if your doctor merely tells you to quit smoking without offering help or support. There are many things that the doctor can do to help you quit. There are medications that decrease craving, programs to help you stop, hypnotherapy, and supplements, which ease the discomfort of withdrawal. Cigarette smoking is extraordinarily addictive and very difficult to stop. You deserve help. A doctor who won't offer that help is not serving you properly.

Don't let a physician make you feel ashamed of a condition that threatens your health, or intimidate you in such a way that you are afraid to ask for help with a problem. If that is the kind of relationship you have with your doctor, find someone who not only specializes in your problem and is therefore better equipped to give you answers, but who is also more proactive and compassionate.

Chapter 21

Making Sense of Your Symptoms

The first question to ask yourself, as you become your own health care advocate, is this: Am I in good health now? How do I find out? There are many ways to do that. If you now have a great relationship with a general practitioner or internist who functions as your "family doctor," approach him or her with the idea that you want to start your own medical record at home (as detailed in Chapter 15). It would contain copies of all relevant past lab reports, consultations, procedure findings, and office notes so that you will always have it with you in case you visit a specialist or an alternative health care practitioner. Then ask for his or her opinion of your general health. Is there anything that looks like a chronic condition and needs closer attention?

If you are experiencing any symptoms but are uncertain what type of HCP to see, perhaps you should do a little reading. I found a very interesting website, www.diagnose-me.com, which has an exhaustive 900+ set of multiple choice questions about your health, diet, medications, and supplements, and asks minute details about everything from the shape of your toenails to the texture of your hair and everything in between. When you are finished filling out the questionnaire, you get three choices: the first and least expensive is a multiple-page computer analysis listing an extensive differential diagnosis of every symptom you have, along with a percentile probability for each. It costs $25 for a complete computer analysis. For $47, a doctor of your choice from the website's list (which includes naturopaths, chiropractors, and M.D.'s) will spend 15 minutes reviewing your results and make a brief comment. Of course, there is the deluxe version for $77, which gives a more thorough overview by the doctor of your choice, whom you can then contact at no additional charge if you have any questions. If you don't want to pay anything at all, the website will still provide you a health overview ("just the headlines") based on your questionnaire, without charge.

I tried this out at the $77 rate and received an 81-page report! I was pretty spooked by the mention of "ovarian cancer" about 10 times, but for anyone in my age group with a checked complaint of abdominal discomfort, any doctor should rule out the fastest growing and most deadly condition that could explain many vague abdominal complaints. Other than that, there were a lot of interesting observations. The doctor's note was two pages long and tried to prioritize the feedback in terms of what possible diagnoses I might want to look into first. I am sure if I were not a physician I would be on the phone in a hot minute asking about this "ovarian cancer" thing, so for most people the extra $30 for telephone access to the doctor might be well spent.

Other websites provide similar "expert systems" questionnaires to help you determine if you have a specific condition. For example, I went to Google and typed in "what are the causes of migraine headaches?" I was taken to a list of sites (many of them advertisements for prescription medications), and as I went down the list, I found a Question and Answer session with a migraine specialist on WebMD that asked and answered (from a traditional medical viewpoint) just about anything you would want to know to differentiate a migraine from a tension headache. There was also an explanation of why pain pills aren't always the best answer, and what the other treatment options are for migraine.

Going back to Google, I entered "Natural remedies for migraine headaches" and found several sites, some offering naturopathic remedies and analysis, others suggesting homeopathic remedies or acupressure and massage techniques. I read a research article that said magnesium relieved migraines in 50 percent of subjects in a double-blind study, compared to 58 percent who took 100 mg of Imitrex™, the most prescribed acute migraine medication in the United States. (Unfortunately, nearly one in five of them got diarrhea as a side effect, and apparently this was less tolerable to patients than the dizziness, sedation, and chest and face tingling sensations in the Imitrex™ treated group.) There are forms of magnesium, like magnesium glycinate, that don't cause diarrhea. This form of the mineral was apparently not used in the study.

If you looked up "fatigue," "joint pain," or "insomnia" and followed the trails you would find similar information that either did or did not fit your set of symptoms and could help you aim for the right sort of health practitioner.

If you are really interested in exploring your health, and you have a PDA (a Palm, Treo, iPaq, iPhone or some handheld computerized notebook) you might be interested in investing in Epocrates™ (www.epocrates.com). The previously mentioned software subscription service allows you to download a rather extensive reference system for prescription medicines and commonly used herbal/vitamin treatments. It also has available a "full package" that includes a symptom-based system: you input the age, gender of the person in question, and duration of the problem, and then start listing all the symptoms. When you hit "go," you will get a list of possible medical conditions, in order of likelihood, which could cause all the symptoms.

There is another section called DX (diagnosis) that allows you to input a disease or condition, and Epocrates™ will generate a brief description of that illness, what tests could be performed to confirm the diagnosis, and what treatment options there are in the current "standard of care." Alternative medicine options are not included. There is also a lab section into which you can program your lab results and learn what they mean, what the "normal range" is, and what problems can cause a "high" or "low" result on that test. You can also look up drug-drug and drug-herb interactions, a very useful feature.

Epocrates™ proved useful to one patient who came to see me for a list of complaints that included ringing in the ears (tinnitus), severe fatigue, weight gain, new onset of binge eating (but no weight loss when patient controlled binge eating for two months), memory problems, and nightmares. He was taking Zoloft and Depakote for bi-polar disorder. He said the Depakote was fairly recently added and helped tremendously with his irritability.

When the patient tried to stop Depakote, his irritability came back. The drug is an anti-convulsant (used for seizures) but is also commonly prescribed for migraine control and mood disorders. He had never tried any other mood stabilizers for his irritability, nor had his psychiatrist mentioned that other possibilities existed. He was just cautioned not to try stopping his Depakote again. It turns out that all of the symptoms for which he came to see me are listed as common side effects of Depakote. When the dosage was increased, his symptoms worsened. These possible side effects were never mentioned to the patient, and alternatives to Depakote were not offered, even after he complained of the symptoms.

I showed him the list of common side effects of Depakote on my version of Epocrates™. I also enlightened him about the probability that another medicine might be as effective in controlling his mood disorder, without causing the side effects. This one single piece of knowledge of how to find out about drug interactions and side effects helped this man become a powerful patient. So many of us do not feel that we are entitled to question a prescribing doctor, or we don't know where to look for information we can use in questioning the doctor.

Now you know!

The more you know about your symptoms, the more informed you will be when discussing them with your consultant. You may even discover that there are some treatments you could try on your own, before seeking a medical appointment. For example, there are many herbal treatments for allergies that are very effective in tackling "hay fever" (a.k.a allergic rhinitis), and you may find one of these works just great for you, without waiting to see an allergist, an ear, nose, and throat specialist, or even your family doctor.

Once you have a good idea of what your symptoms, are, and what they "might" mean, you are prepared to consider your options for a consultation. If from everything you have read, your symptoms are serious and may indicate an urgent problem, you should try to "rule out" that problem first.

Let's say you were in your local pharmacy and took advantage of the free blood pressure machines that are often near the prescription pick-up window. You sit down, slide your arm in, and push the button. Your blood pressure read-out is 270/130 and it is blinking. This is a very high blood pressure. Does this mean you are about to have a stroke?

First, you will want to know if anything is wrong with the blood pressure machine. (People with large arms often register higher BP's because the cuff is too small for them). Ask the pharmacist if there is a problem with the machine; and if you don't know if your arm is too big for the machine, ask. If you had trouble comfortably fitting your arm in, it probably is too tight and will read too high. Try the machine again, after relaxing in the chair a bit. If it is high again, and the cuff isn't too tight, you should contact a doctor right away. Most of the time, high blood pressure does not have symptoms, but can cause very serious problems, such as a stroke, especially if you also have high cholesterol, diabetes, are overweight, or have problems breathing.

We can't possibly cover all the symptoms that you should take seriously, but I will list a few of the important ones:

A change in weight (either up or down) that is not explained by different eating habits. If you have lost your appetite and are losing a lot of weight, you should check it out. Likewise, a sudden weight gain, especially if you have not changed your diet or activity level, can also be a possible "danger" sign.

Breathing problems, of any kind. If you find it difficult to catch your breath, feel you have to "push" to get air in or out of your lungs, have breathing problems with mild exertion or with a change in position (such as lying down), or you seem to run out of breath while talking, these are all signs that you have a problem that needs addressing. It could be an allergy, an infection, the side effect of a medicine you are taking, or a heart or lung problem. Breathing difficulty, whether from coughing, wheezing, or just 'catching" your breath, should never be ignored. Perhaps you will be told that you need to lose weight. That is the simple explanation, but if your weight is such that you become breathless carrying yourself around, you should not accept just a finger wagging from the doctor. You need help losing weight because this symptom has reached crisis level. Other causes of breathlessness include asthma, obstructive lung disease (there are several types), and fluid in the lungs. A weakened heart and some medications can cause it too. The worst-case cause is tumors. Not only is lung cancer a high incidence cancer, but also the lungs filter blood from all organs. As the red blood cells are channeled through the lungs to exchange Co_2 (carbon dioxide) for oxygen, so are cancer cells from other organs. If they break free, they are often "deposited" here or in the liver (another filter for all the blood), and then they grow. You don't have to be a smoker to get lung cancer. Second hand smoke is just as dangerous, and there are lung cancers that are not related to smoking.

Chest pain. Everyone may think they know the description of a heart attack—crushing chest pain, sweating, and shortness of breath—but this is not the only way that a heart attack can present. Many people have described the pain, after it has proven to be a heart attack, as "indigestion," "a sharp pain," "uncomfortable pressure," or just a feeling of weakness and heaviness in the left arm. Months before someone has a heart attack, he/she may be experiencing "angina," which is chest pain of a similar nature that seems to go away with rest. Just because it goes away does not mean that you don't have something serious. You should always have chest pain evaluated. Chest pain can be caused by problems with the esophagus (where the food travels to the stomach from the mouth), problems in the lungs, diaphragm, or the muscles of the chest or the ribs.

Masses. A "mass" is something you can feel that wasn't there before. It could be a lump or bump in breast tissue, the belly, your skin, your armpit, groin, scrotum, or vagina. If you see a mole that changes color, has an irregular border, or feels hard, that should be looked into as well. The first worry is cancer, and the sooner you rule that out, the safer you will be. Early cancer is often curable. Ignoring a growing mass can be very dangerous. Cysts are usually not cancer but can be felt as a "mass." They should be evaluated if they are new or have changed in size. A swollen lymph node sometimes feels like a cyst under the skin. It might mean an infection in that vicinity, but could also be something more serious.

<u>Loss of sensation, strength, or use of any part of your body, even temporarily</u>. If a part of your body becomes numb, your hearing or vision changes, or you are unable to walk steadily, it is important to consult a physician.

<u>Pain</u>. This symptom encompasses many different issues. Our sensory nerves send uncomfortable "wake-up" calls to us to take action. The occasional pinch or ache that is inconsistent is probably not dangerous, but pain that won't go away or increases over time in intensity should be investigated. Many doctors, if they cannot explain or treat pain, automatically become suspicious that the patient is angling for narcotic pain medications. Don't be surprised if you get this reaction, but don't continue with a consultant who doesn't believe you and won't take your symptoms seriously. This is also a situation when you would want to review the chart notes, as the doctor may write some inappropriate "opinion" in the chart.

<u>Decreased function</u>. Despite what many HCPs may tell you, if you are not functioning as well in some areas of your life as you had previously, there probably *is* something you can do about it. Whether this is decreased memory, sex drive, and/or performance, agility, or strength, do not ignore it. If it is a function you would rather not "do without," start searching for someone who can help improve that function. There are many weak and frail older people out there, but there are also strong, vital, and healthy ones. If you want to be in the second group, don't settle

for the "give up" message that many health care providers give you.

Headache or pain behind the eyes. There are many causes for headaches, and several very important organs in your head that you don't want damaged by ignoring this symptom or "numbing" it with pain relievers. Some possibilities include (from worst case to least): aneurysm, tumor, stroke, hematoma, high blood pressure, infections, artery inflammation, sinus or middle ear infections (mold, fungus, bacteria or virus), allergies, and increased muscle tension in jaw and in muscles at temples and back of the neck (a.k.a tension headache).

Weakness and fatigue. Everyone can be tired. Not getting enough sleep can cause fatigue and actually increase risk of several illnesses. But even with enough sleep, some people feel a deep sense of physical and mental weariness that goes beyond just feeling tired and is not relieved by a good night's rest. There are many, many causes of weakness and fatigue: hormonal changes, vitamin deficiencies, anemia, infections, neurological problems, circulation problems, sleep apnea, or depression, which can be a type of endocrine/neurological problem that has as much, or more, to do with physical and mental energy than it does with the mood. (It is unfortunate that some people believe depression is a shameful condition that should be kept under wraps. In fact, it is a treatable and, in many cases, curable illness.)

Chronic insomnia. Probably one of the biggest moneymakers in America is treatment for insomnia. We spend more money on sleep aids of all kinds than on almost any other medication. Not only do we buy medicines , herbs and tonics, but also mattresses, pillows, magnets—just about anything we can find to get a good night's sleep. That doesn't include the substances we use to attempt to "unwind" and help us fall asleep, such as alcohol.

Chronic insomnia can increase the risk for many conditions, such as cancer and heart disease. Sometimes, and this is not true for everyone, the issue might be what we must take away or stop doing in order to have better sleep, instead of adding something. However, careful analysis of chronic insomnia is important.

Bleeding. If you have excessive bleeding during menstruation, or start bleeding after menopause, you should be evaluated, not only for the cause of the bleeding but for anemia as well. Your body recycles iron from red blood cells to re-use in making new blood cells. If you lose a lot of blood, your iron stores can become depleted and you will not have enough to make more hemoglobin, hence you will be anemic, which can be felt as fatigue and shortness of breath. Another source of bleeding for both men and women is intestinal bleeding. You might notice this in the stool, mostly as blood mixed in with the stool (while in the small intestine or high in the large intestine), coating the stool (from rectal and anal bleeding), or as black stool (most likely blood from the stomach, blackened by stomach acid). Sometimes intestinal bleeding can be slow enough that it is not visible in the stool. Vomiting what looks like coffee grounds is also a sign of stomach or duodenal ulcer. Vomiting bright red blood is more likely from your esophagus. All of these are serious and need treatment right away. In addition to the above list, there are several other conditions that cause a loss of red blood cells over time, without actual "bleeding." One such example is an infection with Babesia, a protozoan (single celled) organism contracted from an insect bite (usually a tick) that lives in and destroys red blood cells over time and can result in anemia, fatigue, headaches, night sweats, and weakness.

These are only a few of the indications that mean you should seek medical advice. There are lots of other reasons to go to see a health care provider. Any time you think your health is not optimal, even if you believe you know the reason, it is a good idea to do some research on the symptoms you are experiencing to find out if they can be reversed. It may be that you will hear some things you already know, but you might also discover possible solutions that you had not considered, or some compelling reasons to take a corrective action.

Chapter 22

How to Find a HCP That's Right for You

What kind of HCP (health care provider) should you choose for yourself? Getting a basic "Jack or Jill of all trades" primary provider, one whom you trust, is a good start. This would be someone who could do your annual physical examination, order routine lab tests, and would be available on short notice to treat acute conditions. Your next task would be to make sure you have an understanding with this PHP (primary health care provider) that you want on-going access to your chart, as well as copies of all consultations and lab reports. Explaining your goal of keeping an up-to-date, complete personal medical record will, I hope, not only impress your PHP but also convince him or her to help you achieve this. And what about the alternative practitioners I have been referring to throughout the book? Would one of them be right for you?

You will have to first consider which types of health care are most suited to your personal needs and preferences, since, as I already exposed in this book, there are many philosophies of treatment. Some are more appropriate for certain conditions than others, so having a somewhat broad understanding of what is available to you, and what best suits your beliefs and temperament, is important.

First, let's talk about the different healing orientations of health care providers, and how they are likely to interact with you based on their educational background. Not all HCPs fit neatly into these boxes, because there are many who have learned a great deal outside of their specialty training and offer a different approach than the "traditional' practitioner in their field. You can find out this information from the HCP's receptionist before you make an appointment, or by talking to the practitioner, or many times by visiting their website (if they have one).

Here is a brief tutorial to help you in your search:

ALLOPATHIC PHYSICIANS

The term "allopathic" means "*not the same as pathogen*" and refers to the treatment modality. Basically, it means that allopathic doctors use remedies whose effects differ from those produced by the disease. Simply put, we know allopathic doctors as M.D.'s. These physicians look primarily at symptoms and disease processes, and prescribe treatments and interventions to change or eliminate the symptom. Infections are treated with anti-infective agents, such as antibiotics, antivirals, or antifungals; inflammation is treated with Cox1 and Cox2 inhibitors (non-steroidal anti-inflammatories like aspirin, ibuprofen, Alleve™, and Celebrex™) and corticosteroids like prednisone. Surgery is used when deemed necessary for acute, severely invasive, or inflammatory conditions. M.D.'s rely primarily on medications produced by the standard pharmaceutical companies, and most believe that if the drug has not been proven effective in a *double-blind placebo-controlled trial*, then it lacks certain validity. If M.D.'s did not rely on pharmaceuticals promoted by double-blind placebo-controlled studies, many of their colleagues would accuse them of not practicing *evidence-based medicine*. While there is some debate within the allopathic community on this point, by far the majority endorses this stance and practice accordingly.

Both medical doctors and osteopathic doctors prescribe conventional medications, and therefore the pharmaceutical industry is very involved with their education. Both are required to participate in continuing education to earn Continuing Medical Education (CME) credits, and must report attendance at these educational conferences when they renew their medical licenses every two to three years, according to the requirements in each state. Not surprisingly, pharmaceutical companies put a lot of money into sponsoring educational events, speakers, and prominent product displays. There is an incredibly strong bias at these conferences, with the focus on presentations toward newly patented, recently released medications or ones with a long patent life. Physicians almost never hear presentations on generic drugs and nutritional products or lifestyle issues. Pharmaceutical representatives visit the office of every physician, offering free samples of the top selling prescription drugs, and presenting research articles to reinforce the preferred use of their product over the competition's. With this much campaigning directed at the physician, it is not surprising that their views are influenced by the pharmaceutical industry. That is not to say that prescription medications are bad. Many are invaluable and have saved millions of lives.

The caution I put forth here is simply because most of the big money is behind big, drug-driven medicine, and the alternatives are often not seen by the predominant health care providers. This relationship between M.D.'s and the pharmaceutical industry dates back to the founding of the AMA in 1847, as a means of promoting "scientific medical treatment" and discouraging "drugless healers." It has evolved into the gigantic organization it is today. In your search for a HCP, you can opt for practitioners of mainstream treatment, and you can look at some other possibilities. It doesn't hurt you to consider all the options.

Additionally, there are many M.D.'s and D.O.'s who have practices that do not rely entirely on the standard medical model. These HCPs have have changed their orientation to one with a more holistic focus and would be considered complementary or alternative health care providers. It isn't the degree, but the philosophy of the practitioner that determines how they practice, and what they choose to learn beyond what they were taught in medical school.

CHIROPRACTIC PHYSICIANS

Chiropractic is a medical system based on the theory that disease and disorders are caused by a misalignment of the bones, especially in the spine, that obstructs proper nerve functions. Chiropractic was founded in the United States in 1895, when Daniel David Palmer proposed his theory that subluxations of the spine cause many health problems, and that correcting them with adjustments could cure a number of diseases.

Chiropractic medicine has always maintained a certain independence from mainstream medicine. In the late 1890's, Dr. Palmer defied a movement to license health care practitioners by insisting that chiropractic treatments were not medical by nature. He maintained that because his students did not prescribe medications or test blood or urine, they did not require training in medical treatments. Palmer's stand caused him to run afoul of the AMA, which became more powerful in the early 1900's. As a result, he was twice arrested for misrepresenting chiropractic as medical treatment and for practicing osteopathy without a license. His son B.J. Palmer carried on the battle to win recognition for the chiropractic treatment, arguing that it was not a modality for the diagnosis and treatment of disease, but an effective treatment for disorders of the musculoskeletal system.

Today there is still controversy as to the extent of benefit, but chiropractic schools are now regulated and licensed. Chiropractic physicians attend their chiropractic medical schools, just like M.D.'s and D.O.'s, and extensively study human anatomy and physiology, especially as it relates to blood flow, lymphatic drainage, and nerve function. They learn a very sophisticated method of diagnosing and treating the spine and all the movable parts of the body, as well as attend to proper blood flow through muscles. They learn to read X-rays, not only as a radiologist does, looking out for changes in the bones and joints, but also for the relationship of one bone to another when at rest and in various positions. Their understanding of these mechanics of posture, movement, and alignment help them to make adjustments in the spine, hips, and other areas to return them to optimal position for decreased pain, maximal movement, strength, and body function. Practitioners are also taught diagnosis of more serious conditions, so that appropriate referrals can be made in a timely manner to the correct specialist.

Many chiropractors work with nutritional supplements as well. Some of the chiropractic schools provide extensive training in nutritional therapies and exposure to other disciplines, such as Oriental Medicine and acupuncture, while others don't, and chiropractic doctors continue to receive training in nutritional medicine at conferences after graduation. Chiropractors cannot prescribe pharmaceutical medications, but they can order blood tests in some states, and can order X-rays and physical therapies, as well diagnostic tests of urine and saliva.

Take California chiropractors Ellen Hoffman and John Moore. Before Ellen became a chiropractic doctor, she was a patient herself. As she tells it, "I had a ski injury that put me in the hospital when I was 19 and left me with horrible back pain and chronic kidney, bladder, and menstrual discomforts and infections. I was a wreck for eight years. A few years later, I got in a car accident that left me with a neck injury—for four years, I would carry my neck around at the end of the day by wrapping it in a towel and supporting it with my hand. Then two years after that, I got a tailbone ski injury. I finally went to a chiropractor at the urging of a friend. At that time I was a high school science teacher, but when I recovered fully I decided to become a chiropractor."

What is Ellen's approach to a patient? "First I look at the general neurology of the person," she says, "Neurology is housed in the bone structure; it comes out the brain and down the spinal cord. If there are any misalignments of the spine, they are going to affect the neurology. And I check functional neurology to see if a patient has normal gait patterns. I do something called applied kinesiology, which is a muscle testing technique, and I can evaluate if a muscle turns on when it's supposed to turn on. Then I can find out where the primary problems in the body are. I individually palpate every vertebra to see if they're working right. After that, I use specific techniques to improve bone alignment, reduce stress and tension on joints and vertebrae, and decrease pain. All the work I do is to support normal physiology and remove interferences so that the body can heal itself."

John Moore is Ellen's husband and partner. He is a licensed chiropractor and has post-graduate training in sports medicine and clinical nutrition. "It takes four years to get certified as a chiropractor, after you go through your undergraduate education, and it takes about as many hours as medical school—about 5,200 to 5,500 hours," he says. "Then you do your specialties on top of that: my sports training degree was a one year program; my clinical nutrition training was a three year program."

John and Ellen's practice is holistic in approach, offering not only their own skills, but also bringing in other professionals to support improving health through lifestyle, fitness, and stress reduction. "We offer massage therapy, chiropractic, clinical nutrition, and we also have a person who does stretching classes and Pilates-based classes, as well an acupuncturist."

This is John's take on how alternative or natural medicine is different from the typical, traditional medical practice: "With natural health care, which is in many ways geared more toward eastern philosophies, you don't necessarily treat the disease, you treat the person," he says. "If you come in with insomnia, for example, we might run a series of biochemical tests and we might find a whole array of things to treat you for biochemically that would differ from the next person who comes in with insomnia. If you go to a medical doctor, he or she would typically say, 'Take Ambien.' They'll give very similar medications to people with the same symptoms. However, someone who is 21 and male may be very different biochemically from someone who's 45 and female. You have to look at the individual. And I think that's one of the huge strengths of alternative health care: we *do* look at the individual rather than just saying you're a 'named' disease."

Does chiropractic work? Deborah Bernardi certainly thinks so. She is an English Language and Literature Professor at Carroll College in Helena, Montana. She has suffered from back problems for many years and has tried just about every treatment she could find. While Deborah was in graduate school, her mother (in New Jersey) recommended the chiropractor that she was seeing. This doctor gave her some very useful advice over the phone about how to stand and sleep, to take pressure off her most painful areas, and where to apply ice. This doctor suggested that she find a local chiropractor, and Deborah decided to give it a try. "When you are in pain, you will look for anything that might help," she says.

After only three visits to the chiropractor, she felt a noticeable improvement, and after a while, she didn't need pain medicine at all. She was able to walk and sit for hours without pain. "At that point I decided chiropractors were helpful and decided to see them in the different places where I've lived during my life," Deborah reports." Now she sees a chiropractor only when she experiences pain, which might be two or three times a year, and typically she feels better in one or two sessions.

To find a chiropractor near you, I suggest visiting www.chirodirectory.com, as it not only helps you locate a chiropractor, but also gives you information on what kinds of techniques they have been trained in, along with the definition of those techniques. Of course, the best source is a trusted friend or a relative who has a personal positive experience with a practitioner. That doesn't necessarily mean that you will, but it is less of a "blind" choice.

HOMEOPATHIC PHYSICIANS

Homeopathy is a complementary disease treatment system in which a patient is given minute doses of substances that in larger doses would produce symptoms of the disease itself.

The basic principle of many homeopathic treatments is that our bodies will correct imbalances naturally, on their own, and when they don't, only a "hint" of a direction is needed to help the body correctly adapt and return to balance, or *homeostasis*. Thus, if a person has a headache, a homeopathic remedy might be a minute amount of a substance that would cause a headache if given in a large dose, but the dose is so small it has no direct effect on its own. It is postulated that the system will react to the stimulus of the homeopathic dose and produce its own remedy for the headache.

Despite criticism from the mainstream medical community, the number of homeopathic practitioners and people who use their services has been growing. In fact, there are many instances where the homeopathic approach is valid and gets results. Unfortunately, not many studies are published on homeopathic treatments, especially comparing them to other treatments for similar conditions. Still, there have been several reviews of homeopathic research in medical literature, and in 1997, the reputable medical journal, *The Lancet*, published an article reviewing studies showing that homeopathic treatment was 2.45 times more effective overall than placebo. Later reviews, such as were again reported in *The Lancet* in 2005, were less friendly and suggested that there was essentially no difference between placebo and homeopathic remedies. However, the popularity of homeopathic treatments, especially for infants, children, and even pets (who are unlikely to have a placebo response) has grown. In Europe, as many as 45 percent of physicians have referred patients to a homeopathic practitioner or have prescribed homeopathic remedies themselves. Homeopathic remedies are sold over the counter because they are non-toxic, and you do not have to be a licensed physician to prescribe them, though many homeopathic practitioners are. The FDA does regulate homeopathic remedies to confirm that they contain exactly what they advertise.

NATUROPATHIC PHYSICIANS

For the definition of naturopathic medicine I went to the Dictionary of Occupational Titles of America and found a pretty thorough quote:

"Diagnoses, treats, and cares for patients, using system of practice that bases treatment of physiological functions and abnormal conditions on natural laws governing human body: Utilizes physiological, psychological, and mechanical methods, such as air, water, light, heat, earth, phytotherapy, food and herb therapy, psychotherapy, electrotherapy, physiotherapy, minor and orofacial surgery, mechanotherapy, naturopathic corrections and manipulation, and natural methods or modalities, together with natural medicines, natural processed foods, and herbs and nature's remedies. Excludes major surgery, therapeutic use of x-ray and radium, and use of drugs, except those assimilable substances containing elements or compounds of body tissues and are physiologically compatible to body processes for maintenance of life."

In my experience, naturopathic physicians are thoroughly trained in botanical medicine, as well as in human physiology. They could just as easily be natural medicine pharmacologists, able to compound their own medicines, as well as sit with a patient and evaluate and diagnose a condition. They do not have the right to prescribe pharmaceutical drugs (except in Washington, Oregon, Arizona, and limited rights in California), and many states restrict their herbal prescribing rights as well. Unless a particular state recognizes the naturopathic doctor as qualified to prescribe the medicines that they can make from plants or order from naturopathic apothecaries, it restricts them to practice only a small subset of their skills or to work under the supervision of a licensed medical doctor. This is the case in most states.

The following states license naturopathic physicians: Alaska, Arizona, California, Connecticut, District of Columbia, Hawaii, Idaho, Kansas, Maine, Montana, New Hampshire, Oregon, Utah, Vermont, and Washington. That's 15 out of 50 states, and all but California and D.C. are areas that have a shortage of physicians. If your state isn't listed, and you think you would like to have the option of allowing naturopathic doctors to use the full scope of their training in your state, you can find out how to support legislative change in this direction by visiting this website: www.naturopathic.org/licensure/legislatures_orgs.aspx.

Dr. Michael Bergcamp, a naturopathic physician, a licensed acupuncturist, and Chairman of the Board of Naturopathy in Minnesota, relates a story about studying acupuncture in a hospital in China. After a demonstration by an Oriental Medical Doctor, he expressed through a translator his gratitude to the instructor for showing him this new technique. The Chinese physician laughed and when asked what he found funny, he replied that he had recently read in a Western medical journal about research that concluded that the practice of acupuncture is effective. He found this hysterical, as the practice of acupuncture has been around for 2,000 years and considered highly effective by a large portion of the world's population who have studied it, taught it, and used it to treat many medical conditions.

Dr. Bergcamp thinks that we in the USA are conditioned to believe that we have reached the pinnacle of medicine, but that most of the world does not share our view. Certainly, one sees in the press skepticism about medicine that is not endorsed by the FDA. "This skepticism, in my experience, is one that is self-created by the powerful AMA so that people are continually thinking that CAM [complementary and alternative] medicine is unsafe," he notes.

I asked Dr. Bergcamp what the difference is between his practice and conventional medicine. "What I'm doing is often 'undoing,' this drug miss-practice, the wrong use or the overuse of pharmaceuticals," he says. "And I can't even begin to get a patient better until I've addressed that. Very often I have to start by uncovering a drugged individual, so that we can actually get to his or her health. The core of the conventional medical model, and the big difference between that model and CAM model, is simply this:

We—the naturopathic, alternative medical community—believe that the body is capable of healing itself, and we use many modalities to do that. I know that's rhetoric. Some days I can do that, some days I cannot. But that is the principle difference in our view of the human body and human being that causes the divergence in treatment. The conventional M.D.'s are dealing with disease management. I love how managed care has snuck into the language. 'I'm getting managed care.' What does that mean? It means you are getting disease management. I also think it's a misnomer to say 'health care'. I don't think we have health care in America right now. We have disease management."

All in all, the more choices we have in seeking medical treatment the better off we will be. I have found naturopathic practitioners to be highly knowledgeable and talented individuals. Within the context of their training, they are schooled in Chinese acupuncture and herbology, as well as homeopathic medicine, and extensively trained in counseling, enabling them to advise their patients on the very necessary and difficult issues of lifestyle, habits, and diet.

OSTEOPATHIC PHYSICIANS

This is a system of medicine based on the theory that many diseases are caused by misalignments of bones, ligaments, and muscles and that correcting these anomalies through manipulation can cure the problems. This may sound the same as a chiropractor's job description, but it is not. Osteopathy is as a more complete system of health care than is chiropractic, though D.O. schools do offer classes in a form of manipulation that is similar to chiropractic. The Doctor of Osteopathy's scope of practice in the United States is virtually identical to that of an M.D., though the osteopathic philosophy is more holistic. D.O.'s participate in all medical sub-specialties alongside their M.D. counterparts.

Osteopathic medicine, as practiced and taught in the United States, was established in the late 1800's by Andrew T. Still, M.D. Still worked as an apprentice physician for his father and was employed as a Hospital Steward and Scout Surgeon during the American Civil War. Treating battlefield injuries, and observing the deaths of three children from meningitis in 1864, left him disillusioned with the practice of medicine. He believed traditional medicine to be ineffective at best and harmful at worst and devoted the next ten years to studying the human body and its disorders.

Based on his research, Dr. Still established a medical practice that promoted the philosophy that the human body had the ability to heal itself and that physicians could be taught to remove obstacles to this healing. He believed that physicians should focus not on treating a disease, but on treating the whole patient. He also emphasized preventive medicine and adherence to a healthy lifestyle. In 1892, Still founded this country's first osteopathic school, the American School of Osteopathy in Kirksville, Missouri.

Around 1899, there was a popular movement to get physicians licensed and to have medical schools accredited. There was also a strong push at that time to reduce the ability of the consumer to obtain patent medicines without medical advice, and a strong bias against "drugless healers," which included homeopaths and chiropractors. This is the same campaign that Daniel Palmer resisted, claiming chiropractic physicians should not be subject to the licensing procedures. Dr. Still took a different stance and responded to the pressure to regulate and restrict medical schools by creating credentialing boards in every state where there was an osteopathic school. The schools of osteopathy also included standard medical training for their students, the same training as that provided by schools for allopathic (M.D.) physicians. This met the requirements that were established by the

AMA and thus protected osteopathic medical schools. In licensing, education, and practice, osteopathy became virtually identical to allopathic medicine.

There are philosophical differences, however. An osteopathic physician is taught that it is most important to direct treatment towards assisting the body to heal itself. While manipulative treatments are taught, and research is conducted on the benefits of manipulative treatments at most osteopathic medical schools, the entire curriculum of the standard M.D. medical school is also taught, with an emphasis on integrating all the systems, rather than viewing the body as a series of specialty oriented sections. Below are the principles upon which osteopathic medical practice is based.

Osteopathic principles:

These are the eight major principles of osteopathy that are widely accepted throughout the osteopathic community. They are taken from the curriculum of the Kirksville College of Osteopathic Medicine, a school based on A.T. Still's teachings:

1. The body is a unit.
2. Structure and function are reciprocally inter-related.
3. The body possesses self-regulatory mechanisms.
4. The body has the inherent capacity to defend and repair itself.
5. When the normal adaptability is disrupted, or when environmental changes overcome the body's capacity for self-maintenance, disease may ensue.
6. The movement of body fluids is essential to the maintenance of health.

7. The nerves play a crucial part in controlling the fluids of the body.

8. There are somatic (of or relating to the body) components to disease that are not only manifestations of disease, but also are factors that contribute to maintenance of the disease state.

These principles are not held by osteopaths to be empirical laws, nor contradictions to orthodox medical principles; they are thought to be the underpinnings of the osteopathic perspective on health and disease.

Many osteopaths choose general practice, because it encompasses treatment of all the systems, as they were trained to do. There are, however, specialists of every type, such as neurosurgeons, cardiologists, urologists, and dermatologists, D.O. practitioners who have undertaken osteopathy residencies in these fields. Many D.O.'s, however, have done specialty training at M.D. institutions.

Some osteopathic physicians in the specialties continue to have a whole body approach to patient care, as it is ingrained in the osteopathic medical school curriculum, but many are influenced by the big pharmaceutical companies and follow the same "standard of care" belief and practice as their M.D. counterparts. I am sure the American Osteopathic Association would take issue with me on this, but as a D.O. who believes in the founding principles of osteopathy, and who did specialty training at both M.D. and D.O. institutions, I can see the difference in philosophy and how it alters the way we look at a patient.

To find an osteopathic physician in your area, try www.osteopathic.org/directory.cfm or your yellow pages. You can also ask friends, relatives, and colleagues for a recommendation.

ORIENTAL MEDICINE DOCTORS

I already talked about this specialty at length earlier in this book, but would like to add more information.

There are many types of training that would qualify a person to say that he or she practices Oriental Medicine and acupuncture, though some require more training than others, and licensing is different from state to state.

Here is an overview of the various classes of Oriental Medicine:

> **DIPLOMA**: Practitioner attended school or apprenticeship ranging in time from 16 months to six years. Curricula vary based on the traditions of a particular school and on the length of training. Much of the data accumulated over centuries of Oriental medical practice comes from the teachings and notes of thousands of practitioners over time.
>
> **CERTIFICATE**: Same as Diploma
>
> **M. Ac. (Master of Acupuncture)**: Usually two to three years undergraduate and two years graduate study. No herbal study is required.
>
> **MTCM (Master of Traditional Chinese Medicine)**: Usually two years under-graduate and three to four years graduate study of all methods of Traditional Chinese Medicine.

M.S. OM (Master of Science in Oriental Medicine): Usually two years undergraduate plus three to four years graduate study of all methods of Oriental Medicine.

OMD (Oriental Medical Doctor): Usually five years of school. Now offered only in Asian schools; offered in the U.S. until approximately mid 1980's.

CMD (China Medical Doctor): Medical doctor licensed in Mainland China. Curriculum does **not** include Traditional Chinese Medicine but many CMDs acquire training through in-service education.

There are also Oriental medical doctors who can obtain certification in medical acupuncture, which does not include the use of herbs. The whole philosophy of Oriental Medicine comes from two primary disciplines that have shared knowledge and practices over the course of the 20th century: Korean and Chinese traditional medicine. Both disciplines have very long traditions and histories, dating back to 1,000 BC or further.

In the earliest days of the practice of herbal medicine, there was an exchange of ideas between Indian, Korean, and Chinese practitioners. With wars and territorial isolation, these disciplines developed with some similar roots but had different remedies and diagnostic methods. Still, there are some striking similarities between Oriental and Ayurvedic (i.e. Indian, which we'll discuss in a minute) theory and practice. Both Oriental and Ayurvedic medicine view the whole person as a system that should be in balance, and both schools of thought use herbs, massage, meditation, exercise, and diet as very important ingredients of treatment.

In Japan, Oriental Medicine was most largely influenced by its closest neighbor, Korea, but it also developed some unique characteristics and remedies of its own. For example, Traditional Chinese Medicine generally uses deeper and stronger acupuncture techniques than the Japanese style of acupuncture, which uses finer needles and more superficial puncture techniques. Both use the meridian system for locating acupuncture sites. One source mentioned another difference, which is that Japanese practitioners do not utilize herbal treatments, while Chinese practitioners often combine them with acupuncture treatment.

Oriental Medicine is not only based on the practice of herbal remedies and the use of acupuncture, but also on an entirely different way of viewing human physiology from that of the Western model, which is based on structure, function, and pathogens. Possibly the best way I can describe it is to say that the Oriental medical doctors use methods unique to their own practice to observe a person in much the same way a meteorologist might observe satellite images and weather readings of pressure, wind, and humidity to determine and predict weather. But in the case of Oriental Medicine, the practitioner also works to modify "internal disturbances" so as to re-establish the normal flow of energies, that is, Qi or Chi.

While the Oriental system does identify and name specific organs and functions, it also treats organs that have no specific location in the body, and assigns attributes to organs (such as certain emotional states) in ways that would seem baffling to a Western medical practitioner. Thus, you might hear an Oriental medical doctor talk about a "damp wind in the liver," a "stagnant liver," or a "dry wind in the triple burner." ("Triple burner" refers to an energy system that encompasses the stomach and intestines.)

I have found Oriental Medicine to be particularly helpful when there are multi-system complaints, viral conditions, fatigue, or pain. Visit www.orientalhealthsolutions.com/faq.html for an excellent overview of frequently asked questions about Chinese Medicine and provides links to an extensive search engine for finding a local practitioner certified in both acupuncture and herbology (http://dol.jkmcomm.com/acupuncture/default.asp).

Using the search function, I was able to locate 2,643 practitioners in California, 858 in Colorado, 35 in Arkansas, and 990 in Florida. I didn't search every state, but my results satisfied me that even in places like Arkansas, where alternative medicine is not common, there can still be found some certified practitioners in the larger cities.

AYURVEDIC PHYSICIANS

The practice of Ayurvedic Medicine developed in India and can be traced as far back as 520 BC, during the lifetime of the Buddha. There have been several periods in the history of the Indian subcontinent when the philosophy and practice of Ayurvedic Medicine has blossomed with new knowledge and insights, due to the contributions of individuals who wrote down their principles and practice and to the founding of schools for the study of medicine.

The practice declined when the British, who established a colony in India in 1858, opened their own medical schools and hospitals. After India's independence in 1947, Ayurvedic practice began to become popular again, incorporating not only its traditional concepts, but also many Western and Oriental treatments.

The goal in Ayurvedic practice is to restore harmony to the body, mind, and spirit through the understanding of the basic nature of the individual and the disharmony that may be present. Imbalances are corrected through diet, massage, herbal treatments (both ingested and applied to the skin), and meditation.

A substantial amount of Western research has been conducted into the chemical nature and properties of both Ayurvedic and

Oriental medicines and herbs to determine their active constituents and the specific biochemical actions within the body that account for their effectiveness. Many patented medicines have been developed from this research, as an active component becomes identified and is able to be synthetically derived or copied. I think that most Western herbalists (as well as Oriental and Ayurvedic ones) would say that one single active ingredient extracted from a healing herb does not provide the same benefits as the whole herb.

OTHER MAINSTREAM AND ALTERNATIVE HEALTH CARE PROVIDERS

Nurse Practitioners (NPs) and Physician Assistants (PAs): NPs and PAs are both of the Western medical orientation in their basic training, although some might seek additional post-graduate training in complementary and alternative medicine and offer alternative medical treatments. Both NPs and PAs require extra years of training beyond a bachelor's type, medical-oriented program, which might have earned them a nursing, emergency medical technician, or a laboratory technologist degree. The advanced schooling usually lasts about three years. Upon certification, graduates are qualified to perform physical exams and to provide treatment (including writing prescriptions) under the supervision of a practicing physician. It is common to have the physician do the initial diagnostic evaluation, and then the NP or PA does follow-up care and management. In areas where there is a shortage of doctors, the support of Nurse Practitioners and Physician Assistants is extremely valuable.

Massage Therapists: Don't ever underrate the value of a massage until you have had one from a well trained professional masseuse or masseur. Not only do tired and tight muscles feel better, but also the circulation is improved, and many studies have shown that massage helps elevate the mood and improve the immune system function.

There are as many types of massages as there are medical practitioners, perhaps more. I will outline a few of the more popular ones that you might be able to locate in your area.

Deep Tissue Massage has several subtypes, such as Rolfing, Heller technique, and Myofascial Release. The fascia is the connective tissue "wrapping" around muscles that connect and hold muscle groups together. Thus, if one muscle in the group is in spasm, it affects the function of the whole muscle group. Releasing that tension, with deep, slow, constant pressure along the lines where fascia is interconnecting several muscles, aids in releasing the tension and reducing chronic pain. This can often be done without oils or creams, because the movement is slow, but it can also be done with massage oil. This is not generally considered a "relaxing" massage, as the recipient is not likely to drift off to dreamland when a tender muscle group has pressure applied steadily to it. Experienced practitioners try to keep the pain felt during the treatment to a minimum. The best result is that one feels invigorated and has a greatly improved mobility. It is typical for Rolfing and Heller work to be performed as a "set" of several sessions, typically about ten. The practitioners use their hands, elbows, and forearms as well as the flat of the hand and fingers to get into deep tissue areas.

Eselen Massage, which takes its name from the retreat and conference center on California's Big Sur coastline where its developer taught this practice, has many similarities to the classic Swedish massage, but also includes an emphasis on the emotional rapport between therapist and recipient. In addition to the long soothing strokes of traditional massage, gentle rocking of the body and passive movement of the joints to improve flexibility are included.

Reflexology comes from Chinese medical practice, where it is believed that there are neurological connections between specific areas on the feet and the internal organs. Thus, the foot massage is one modality used to treat a patient with certain ailments. While I could not find any research into the effectiveness of Reflexology or foot massage related to internal organs, I can say, as anyone else might who has enjoyed a good foot massage, that they are both invigorating and relaxing at the same time.

Shiatsu is a traditional Japanese style of massage, from which the similar *Trigger Point Massage* may have evolved. The Shiatsu technique involves using the thumbs and knuckles to stimulate trigger points along the energy meridians that are used in acupressure. The recipient wears light, loose clothing during this massage, and often the massage mat is on the floor. Trigger Point therapy is different in that it focuses on certain points in the body where the highest degree of tension or pain is felt. A skilled practitioner can often find these points by feel and will confirm the location of the problem area when the patient responds to pressure on that spot. Some practitioners will use steady pressure to the body, and some use carbon dioxide injections to alleviate the pain and thus provide relief to the whole muscle.

Swedish Massage, was not, ironically, started in Sweden but was first practiced in Holland, by a Dutch practitioner in the 1800's. Swedish Massage is essentially relaxing in nature, with long smooth strokes applied along the body parts (classically in the direction of the heart to improve circulation). Oil, cream, or lotion is applied to the skin to allow the movements of the hands to be smooth and steady.

Thai Massage should not in any way be confused with the "sex-for-sale" disguised as massage that is offered in downtown Bangkok. Thai Massage is an ancient technique that has some roots in Indian massage but has developed a unique flavor of its own.

The recipient is given clean, loose fitting silk or cotton pajamas and lies down on a massage table that is about the size of a twin bed and about 1 foot off the ground.

The massage usually lasts one to two hours, and the therapist uses just about every part of his/her body to work on the recipient (elbows, hands, knees, and feet), and may even stretch the recipient's back over his or her own back for maximal effect. The Thai technique could be considered a combination of massage and passive yoga, as all limbs are stretched, pulled, and maneuvered for a maximum mobility. The therapy is done in a very methodical manner. Sometime the massage room has many tables in it, and all the massage therapists are doing the same movement with their clients in unison, like a dance. Not only is it very invigorating to receive, it is also very interesting to see. In Thailand, a massage may cost no more than $35 for a two-hour treatment, unless you receive it at a five-star hotel, where it would be more and would very likely incorporate the oils. An online search will locate practitioners of Thai Massage in this country.

There are other types of "manual techniques," such as *Muscle Energy Technique, Myofascial Release, Neuromuscular Therapy,* and *Myoskeletal Alignment,* but I felt that these properly belong in the category of Osteopathic Manipulation and Chiropractic techniques, since they are commonly used by both practitioners in the course of their therapies. There may be massage therapists who have learned some of these techniques, and who perform them well, but as a group, Chiropractors and Osteopaths have developed these methods.

To see if I could find a massage therapist in my area, I used Google™ and typed, "find a massage therapist" into the search engine. I got a long list of websites and visited about 10 of them. Three did not give me good results–one gave me the name of only one practitioner, another gave me a list covering the whole state of California. Four websites, however, offered me at least five or six massage therapists within 10 miles of my home. Some of the websites I visited allowed me to specify what type of massage I was looking for as part of the search, and some described within the websites the type of massage therapy offered. You can do a similar search for your area, but your best bet, as with every type of health practitioner, would be a personal recommendation.

In conclusion, the choice of physician or other provider is one of the most important you will make in your role as a proactive, assertive, informed consumer of health care. It will undoubtedly be a choice you make more than once, as your needs change or as you come to recognize that you deserve the best health care provider out there and decide it is worth the effort it takes to find the right one for you—one whom you trust, who is open-minded and who listens and communicates well with you, one who stays up to date on the most current treatments or knows when your health needs lie beyond his or her practice. In your new role as empowered patient, you will settle for nothing less than this.

Epilogue: Final Words

Books are usually written to inspire, inform, and educate readers. That has been my intent as well.

I have presented, to the best of my professional and personal knowledge and ability, the information I believe is not only useful, but also crucial for every consumer and provider of health care. You, the reader, are free to decide what parts of the book are applicable to your own life, and what information therein can enhance and benefit your health.

Any websites I have mentioned in this book should not be considered as sources of medical advice from me to you, but only as examples of resources and options available to you as a consumer of health care.

Remember: an inquisitive, curious, and critical mind that questions and challenges the status-quo, actively searching for better solutions and alternatives to the commonly accepted but flawed model, is the best weapon a person has. Use it to become your own empowered and wise health care advocate.

Whether or not you will go on to join the growing ranks of renegade patients, I thank you for reading this book and wish you excellent health!

Tedde M. Rinker, D.O.

Appendix

Dr. Rinker's Selected Websites and Books

Websites

Diagnosis:

www.diagnose-me.com A detailed questionnaire (it takes an hour to fill out) will provide you with a detailed analysis of possible health concerns in order of likelihood. For a graduated fee you can have a report of increasing thoroughness and complexity, and the top price gets you a health professional (Your choice of HCP type) to review your report and provide a commentary, and answer questions if you have them. I find it to be an excellent resource.

http://symptoms.webmd.com/default.htm A website sponsored by WebMD, that has a detailed analysis of symptoms and proposes many possible causes, which you can select to get additional information to narrow down the diagnosis. You do not get a report with this one, but it is free. It does not represent alternative treatments, only conventional medical diagnosis and treatments.

Patient rights:

www.hhs.gov/ocr/hipaa You can get a detailed summary of your rights to access your medical records, your right to privacy, and your right to see your chart and to make corrections in your medical record. You can download this as a pdf file to your computer and present it to a health care provider who is resistant to providing access to your records, or to making requested changes.

www.askme3.org Here is a download, a 4-page brochure that simplifies the process of obtaining clear information from health care providers. HCP's are required to make sure you understand what you were told about your condition, what is recommended, and why this recommendation is being made. There are the "3 questions" that this brochure mentions to help guide you in making sure this important part of your healthcare visit is not missed, and also 5 steps or suggestions to help you make sure those three questions are answered to your satisfaction and understanding. One of those suggestions is to bring an advocate (a professional or a friend) who will help you make sure these topics are fully covered to your satisfaction. It can be intimidating to listen to someone speak of your illness in a manner you don't understand, and your own anxiety about your illness can make it harder to understand what is being said to you. This can happen easily to anyone, no matter how intelligent they are.

Supplement quality:

www.consumerlab.com This is a website that requires a $29.95 yearly membership and this gives you access to all of their reviews and testing of nutritional supplements. They have an extensive library of tests, and will compare brands and approve or disapprove them based on whether they have the potency advertised on their label, whether they are bioavailable (dissolve adequately enough to be absorbed) and on whether they have any toxic components (such as lead or pesticide residue). These reviews also often give the cost of a dose or the cost per mg of a dose. Sometimes this is the most surprising news of all! There is a wide variation in cost and potency of supplements even within the same manufacturers. A worthwhile investment if you want to find the best supplements to use.

Research:

www.naturaldatabase.com/home This is the website for the Natural Medicine Comprehensive Database, a subscription service that gives both consumer level and professional level information on natural supplements, vitamins and other herbal remedies. They are cautious about stating effectiveness for herbal treatments, and only do so when they can specifically cite Western type controlled studies, typically placebo controlled studies, which would leave out many studies done in other counties or open label studies. Still it does report what the substance has been used for, what names are used for them other than the one you might have looked up, and notes possible side effects and interactions with drugs. Fees for subscribing are $59 for one year, $109 for two years.

www.prescribersletter.com This website is for prescribing physicians and is published by the same group as the Natural Medicine Database. It is a monthly newsletter giving information about the latest prescription drugs to come on the market, and the "scoop" on whether the advertised claims are realistic or not. The slant is clearly in favor of pharmaceutical interventions and the typical conventional medicine slant is evident. Sometimes it addresses issues that make the general press to prepare prescribing physicians for what their patients might bring up. It typically advises physicians on how to answer queries from patients, and generally discourages use of supplements and vitamins to treat illness or prevent disease. This is also a subscription service, and has a large library of back issues and topics.

http://www.crnusa.org The Council for Responsible Nutrition is an organization of nutritional supplement suppliers, manufacturers and researchers whose purpose is declared thus: "CRN's mission is to enhance and sustain a climate for our member companies to responsibly market dietary supplements and their ingredients by maintaining and improving confidence among consumers, media, government leaders, regulators, healthcare professionals and other decision makers with respect to our members' products." In that vein, you can find excellent responses to newspaper and magazine articles that claim nutritional supplements are dangerous. This website provides thoughtful analysis of these reports and presents an alternative perspective.

www.pubmed.com This website is for the National Library of Medicine and has every article published in a medical journal anywhere in the world for the past 10 years. You can search on a specific topic and view abstracts of most of the articles, although some will not present an abstract, only a title and author. You can enter search words such as "breast cancer and green tea" and you'll get 85 scientific papers cited, or "breast cancer and melatonin" and see 307 articles cited. You can send email to yourself and others with these references, once you find them.

Evaluate doctors:

www.ratemds.com This website allows people to anonymously rate doctors on punctuality, helpfulness, knowledge and overall quality. All medical specialties are included and: also Podiatry, Dentistry, Naturopathy, Psychology, and Chiropractic. Some categories (such as Lyme disease specialists) are listed also, even though it is not a traditional specialty. The great thing about this is that one can assume these are from people who have had first hand experience with the doctor or health care provider. On the down side, *anyone* can place a review, both positive and negative. Treat it like gossip: sometimes it's true and sometimes it isn't. One would be suspicious of reviews that have all 5's (top score) and/or by all 1's (worst score). It would be hard to tell then if these are being padded by the doc and trashed by one or more resentful patients. Be sure to place your own reviews of any HCP you have had a negative or positive experience with: the more real-life, honest evaluations there are on a website like this, the better it will be for everyone, including the doctors who are evaluated. They will learn to take every patient more seriously if a resource such as this can provide anyone who checks with an accurate report card.

General Health Information:

www.mercola.com One of the most popular medical type web-sites on the Internet, Dr. Joseph Mercola's site has a ton of information you will not see elsewhere. He has a strong bias toward healthy living, a clean diet (toxin free, non processed foods, etc) and helps people identify the many sources of toxicity to which we are exposed in our everyday lives. He has recently published a new book, "Take Control of Your Health". This is a great self help book for people who want to use diet, lifestyle and nutrients to achieve health, lose weight and feel great.

www.perlhealth.com David Perlmutter, MD is another well-known physician who was among the first to propose nutritional supplementation and treatment for neurological diseases and to prevent the cognitive decline of aging through nutrients. He has a blog, http://renegadeneurologist.com that is well worth visiting. I find Dr. Perlmutter to be an excellent educator and highly recommend his books, "Raise a Smarter Child by Kindergarten" and "The Better Brain Book".

www.drdharma.com Dharma Singh Khalsa, M.D. was one of the first physicians to say that Alzheimer's disease could be prevented with nutrients. He was laughed at when he first made this assertion, but now there is a consensus of support for this concept, and a good body of medical literature to support it. He is a strong supporter of the use of meditation to improve mental function and health as well. This website gives information of improving brain function, the benefits of meditation, and seminars that are presented by his organization.

www.dockidd.com Parris Kidd, PhD, is a nutritional scientist who speaks all over the country and writes many articles on health management through nutritional approaches. His website gives you free access to the many articles he has written. He is a well-respected scientist and a great teacher.

http://www.webmd.com/ This website is a cornucopia of information. It does have articles by MD's but you can also find articles written by science writers, naturopathic physicians, RN's and most healthcare specialists. It would be a good place to go to get some general information on numerous health topics. There are many blogs by health care writers that you can access through this website.

http://www.functionalmedicine.org Functional medicine is personalized medicine that deals with primary prevention and underlying causes instead of symptoms for serious chronic disease. It is a science-based field of health care that is grounded in the following principles: Biochemical individuality, Patient-centered medicine, Dynamic balance of internal and external factors, Web-like interconnections of physiological factors, Health as a positive vitality and Promotion of organ reserve. This is “whole person” medical practice geared toward helping you be a healthy person rather than treating a disease. You can learn about this new approach to medicine at this website and find health care practitioners in your area who use this approach.

www.worldhealth.net This is the international website for the American Academy of Anti-Aging Medicine, founded approximately 14 years ago and it has been growing by leaps and bounds over these years to be a world wide organization today with thousands of physician members. Their purpose is to support learning and research in finding ways to slow and reverse the progress of the degenerative diseases of aging. Hundreds of articles are posted daily to this website, and there is a doctor referral list available to find a practitioner in your area. The only caution I would advise in using this referral list is that you make sure the physician you select is certified by the American Academy of Anti-Aging Medicine, as any practitioner (and even non-practitioners) can register on this list. Visiting the website of a practitioner listed is one way to find out, or call and ask about their certification.

www.wtsmed.org This website is the Restorative Medicine website, and promotes treatment for a condition where a person may have all the symptoms of hypothyroidism but may have lab testing in the normal range. These symptoms include fatigue, dry hair and skin, constipation, slowed thinking, menstrual irregularities, low body temperature, cold hands and feet, weight gain or inability to lose weight even with diet and exercise. This treatment using herbs and sustained release T3 (liothyronine) has helped many people recover their vitality without having to be on thyroid medications for life.

http://www.cnn.com/SPECIALS/2007/news/empoweredpatient/
Patients all over the United States are beginning to adopt a proactive patient mentality, as exemplified by a CNN news story which appeared on the 4th of July, 2008, and is featured on their website. The story honors six heroic "Empowered Patients" who've had to learn the hard way that you cannot passively accept whatever you get from modern medicine. These six people suffered from such traumas as a wrong and potentially fatal diagnosis (only discovered as untrue when the patient insisted on a second opinion against the advice of her physician), to the death of a young man who should have fully recovered from a fracture but died from a hospital acquired infection, to a physician/author who saw so many medical mistakes causing so much harm and illness that he felt he had to take this story to the people. The six heroes of these stories (in the case of the young man who died, it was his parents) all became activists for patient's rights in their communities, helping others to become more powerful and knowledgeable health care consumers. They were honored by CNN on Independence Day, and I felt it fitting, with our Declaration of Independence for Health Care, to honor them here too, by referring you to the website where you can read about their experiences.

Lyme Disease:

Lyme disease is probably the fastest growing infectious disease in the country, and is spreading all over the world as quickly. There is tremendous controversy among physicians, researchers and health information organizations about the abundance of new cases, about the proper treatment of Lyme disease and about the diagnosis of it. I will list below some websites where you can get a full view of the controversy, to decide for yourself where you stand. If you have the symptoms of Lyme disease, this is an important decision to make.

www.cdc.gov/ncidod/diseases/submenus/sub_lyme.htm This is the Center for Disease Control. They make an attempt to be neutral, but support the Infectious Disease Society of America's point of view about the severity of the epidemic and their recommended treatment guidelines for Lyme disease.

http://www.journals.uchicago.edu/doi/full/10.1086/508667 This website will give you the Infectious Disease Society's view of the Lyme disease epidemic, as well as their treatment guidelines.

www.ilads.org This is the website for the International Lyme and Associated Diseases Society, an organization of healthcare practitioners and researchers who find that Lyme disease is a much more serious condition and who recommend more aggressive and thorough treatment. They have published a response to the IDSA treatment guidelines which can be read at his site: http://www.ilads.org/press_10_07.html .

http://www.lymenet.org/ This is the website of the Lyme Disease Network, a nonprofit organization to support health care practitioners and patients in their battle with Lyme disease. This is a great resource for local Lyme disease support groups. There is also a good library of medical abstracts, legal advice and research information.

http://www.betterhealthguy.com This website is managed by Scott Forsgren, a patient-advocate who is also a prolific writer for several well-respected Lyme-related newsletters and publications. This website is a great first stop and offers a great deal of well-organized, highly informative resources.

www.lymeinfo.net/lymediseasebooks.html & www.lymebook.com These are sites that offer books about Lyme disease, including both traditional and alternative treatments. I don't think there is any one answer yet for chronic Lyme disease, but there is hope for improved health and recovery which must be individualized to each patient, as the response to the infection can be highly varied, from mild distress to severe disability to death.

www.lymememorial.org This website is very persuasive regarding the seriousness of this epidemic, citing that new cases in the United States since 1980 exceed that of HIV/AIDS. This is a very sober view indeed, but worth reading.

http://www.lymememorial.org/National_Statistics.htm This page on the website gives the statistics on the spread of this disease, estimating the number of new cases since 1980 in the United States exceeds 3 million people, using the Center for Disease Control's own estimating criteria.

Chronic Fatigue Syndrome:

Also known as Chronic Fatigue and Immune Deficiency Syndrome, is another chronic illness which has swept the nation. But a syndrome does not identify a cause of the disease. This, along with another epidemic condition, Fibromyalgia, are often misdiagnoses of Lyme disease, hypothyroidism and numerous viral infections. Here are some useful websites to learn more about this condition:

http://www.cfids.org/default.asp This is the Chronic Fatigue Immune Deficiency website, a non-profit organization devoted to education and supporting research into this condition, which may be caused by a huge variety of conditions, listed on this page in the website:
http://www.cfids.org/about-cfids/diagnostic-testing.asp#chart

http://www.mayoclinic.com/health/chronic-fatigue-syndrome This educational website is sponsored by the Mayo Clinic and has a more narrow definition of Chronic Fatigue Syndrome and its treatment. It does however, offer some information which may be useful.

http://www.ncf-net.org/ This is the National CFIDS Foundation, primarily directed to funding research to find causes and cures for this condition. There is a substantial amount of information on the site regarding the research funded by this organization and what they have discovered.

CFIDS Support groups can be found on the internet by looking for local groups directly through Google search words, or through this Center for Disease Control (CDC) site: http://www.cdc.gov/cfs/cfssupport.htm .

Books

Merck Manual 18th Edition by Robert S. Porter and Thomas V. Jones (2006) Every medical student or resident gets this book, the most comprehensive review of symptoms and treatment for every medical specialty. It represents the American conventional medicine view.

Merck Manual of Medical Information, Home Edition, by Mark H. Beers (2004) This version is geared to the average reader and simplifies medical terms into everyday language. It also gives less detail about treatment.

Ageless (2007) and The Sexy Years, (2004) by Suzanne Somers These books are really extended interviews with doctors practicing Anti-Aging medicine, sprinkled with personal anecdotes by Ms. Somers. The topics cover the controversies about hormone replacement in menopause, presenting the bio-identical hormone replacement point of view, and the second book includes Anti-Aging medicine's view of preventing degenerative disease in men and women.

Natural Hormone Balance for Women (2002) by Uzzi Reiss and Martin Zucker. Also by Uzzi Reiss, a more recent edition of similar vein, The Natural Super Woman (written with Y'fat Reiss-Gendell) Uzzi Reiss was one of the very first to write extensively about natural (bio-identical) hormone replacement.

Take Care of Yourself, the Complete Illustrated Guide to Medical Self-Care, by Donald M Vickery, and James F. Fries (2006) This is a down-to-earth guide for general health, helping to determine when to seek medical care and when home remedies will work well enough.

Life Extension Foundation's Disease Prevention and Treatment, by Melanie Segala (2003 edition) A very complete, hefty book covering a broad range of topics with extensive bibliographies. This book is very useful for adults wanting to incorporate herbs and supplements into their health care. It includes conventional medicine and research along with more integrated health care.

Healthy Revolution, What You Really Need to Know to Stay Healthy in a Sick World, by David Brady (2007) Dr. Brady has a functional medicine approach, which includes advice on diet, lifestyle, nutritional supplements and personal well-being as parts of an integrated approach to being well and staying well.

Most Effective Natural Cures on Earth, by Jonny Bowden (2008) This is a very useful book, well researched, giving hundreds of remedies for the most comman maladies facing us today. This book is written for use by the average person who might not be familiar with natural remedies and treatments.

When Antibiotics Fail: Lyme Disease and Rife Machines, by Bryan Rosner (2005) Many people with Lyme disease have been refused treatment or under treated, and find themselves on their own, still sick. This survey of alternative treatments used by thousands who report they recovered is very helpful for Lyme disease sufferers.

Mr. Rosner wrote another book, Top Ten Lyme Disease Treatments, along with James Schaller, M.D., Julie Byers and Michael Huckleberry. This combines conventional medical treatments with alternative treatments as a broad consensus of remedies that show promise in healing from Lyme disease (2007)

Healing Lyme: Natural Healing and Prevention of Lyme Borreliosis and Its Coinfections, by Stephen Buhner (2005) Stephen Harrod Buhner has published several books on herbal medicine, and this one has one of the best researched overviews of how people get infected with Lyme disease, and why it is so difficult to diagnose and treat. It also offers a sensible herbal protocol to address the illness. It may not work for everyone, but many have found this treatment successful.

Adrenal Fatigue: The 21st Century Stress Syndrome, by James L. Wilson and Jonathan Wright (2002) This book gives and excellent overview of a condition that is increasingly recognized as contributing to most ill health in our society. Many medical conditions are either caused or made worse by the failure of our adrenal system to maintain a normal resilience and protection from stress.

The Feel-good Guide to Fibromyalgia and Chronic Fatigue Syndrome by Lynette Bassman (2007) Written by a clinician and a former sufferer of CFIDS, it gives a wide array of options to improve health and energy and reduce pain. This book includes both conventional medical approaches and alternative remedies.

www.ingramcontent.com/pod-product-compliance
Lightning Source LLC
LaVergne TN
LVHW011221080426
835509LV00005B/249

* 9 7 8 0 9 7 6 3 7 9 7 7 5 *